158 MUST-KNOW NATURAL & HERBAL REMEDIES FOR (ALMOST) EVERYTHING

158 MUST-KNOW NATURAL & HERBAL REMEDIES FOR (ALMOST) EVERYTHING

Volume 1

Simple Beginner-Friendly, Easy-to-Follow **Organic Recipes**
for Your Family's Health & Wellness

JENNI REMPEL

For Leah & Kailey. Thank you for letting me be your Nana. Grandpa and I are excited to see all the amazing and wonderful things you accomplish so we can be your cheerleaders. We love you, girls!

TABLE OF CONTENTS

OTHER BOOKS BY JENNI REMPEL

Forget The Pharmacy - Grow Your Own Medicine
Grow Your Own Herbal Pharmacy

The Comprehensive Herbal Handbook (2 In 1)

The Herbalist's Healing Garden

The Homesteader Herbal Handbook

SPANISH
El Manual Completo De Hierbas Medicinales (2 En 1) El Manual De
Hierbas Del Hortelano

Olvidate De La Farmacia – Cultiva
Tu Propia Medicina

GERMAN
Vergessen Sie Die Apotheke –
Pflanzen Sie Ihre Eigene Medizi

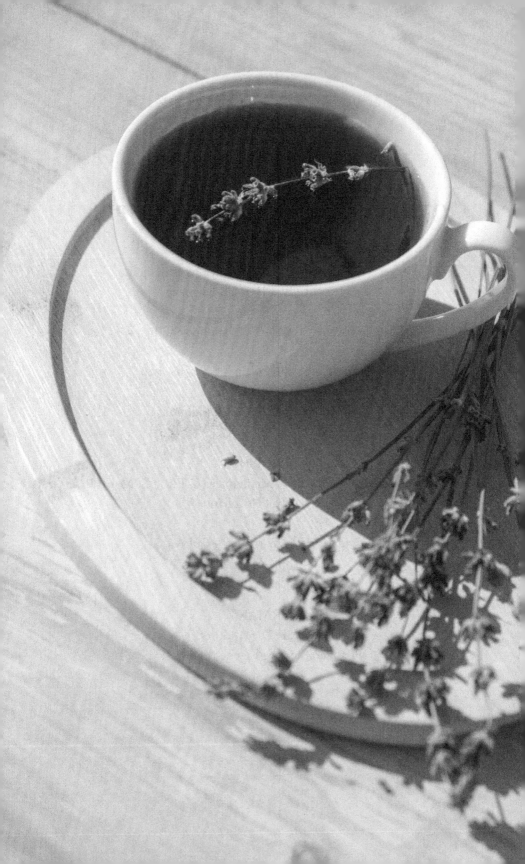

INTRODUCTION

Nature is wonderful. Nature can help you. Nature can nurture you. Wouldn't it be so simple if nature gave us a recipe book of different herbal remedies? For those of us who are looking for ways to stay natural and choose healthy ingredients to boost our health and well-being, a recipe book of some amazing natural remedies is just what we need. And here it is. You are about to learn 158 different and easy-to-create herbal recipes you can try at home.

If you believe that nature holds the power to help us keep our health, if you want to embrace a holistic lifestyle, or you are simply inquisitive about how things work – you have come to the right place.

This is a very practical book. If you have a cold or the flu, go to that chapter and try some of the remedies – You might be surprised how good they make you feel. Have a headache? Check out that chapter and experiment with some wholesome ingredients and easy-to-follow instructions. Struggle with urinary tract infections? Check out some of those recipes too. See which recipes become your favorites.

There are handy symbols for each remedy to make it simple to follow. Each herbal recipe is broken down as follows:

 Medicinal Properties – Learn about what each remedy contains and why it works.

Fun Fact – Learn an interesting fact about the remedy ingredients

 Why Will It Help – Learn what makes this recipe effective

 How to Make It – Find a list of the ingredients and instructions on how to prepare the remedy.

 How to Use It – Learn how to use the remedy

You won't find every ingredient in your kitchen – but many of them are! For the less common ingredients, your local health food store is a great place to start. I have also had good luck ordering ingredients on Amazon.

WHY HERBAL REMEDIES?

For centuries, people have experimented with plants and herbs to find those natural ingredients that promote health. There were no pharmacies and no doctors as we know them today. There was simply trial and error. How courageous those historical experimenters were! I imagine not every experiment was successful. But thank goodness they kept going. Those early learnings became the basis of our modern medical advancements.

As powerful as it is, nature comes with many perks. It can heal us, and it can make us feel better. A part of that healing process are millions of different plants. What is more, some of them are known to have incredible benefits to human health.

These are a part of the herbal medicine. It is a practice that comes from ancient times, and it involves using plants to enhance general well-being. They provide medicinal benefits which are excellent for the overall health of the human body. Some of these plants are so powerful that they must be taken extremely carefully – the same level as you do with some pharmaceutical medications. To understand that, look at some of the medicines you have at home – can you see that most of them are based on versions of naturally occurring compounds found in plants? That should give you the answer you are looking for.

In this book, you will discover 158 different herbal recipes. Some of them can be used to promote overall health, and others can be used to get relief from certain symptoms and health conditions. For those of you who are just dipping your toes into herbal remedies, get ready because there is a lot for you to learn here.

We will explore all types of herbal remedies, starting from ones that will help your digestive system, skin, and respiratory health. There are also recipes for ingredients that are known to boost your immune system and support cardiovascular & urinary tract systems, bones, muscles, ligaments, and even help diabetes!

But don't feel intimidated – as we will start together from the very beginning. Within the first chapter, you will learn how to make all the natural remedies in your home. Whether you want to learn how to make a tincture, tea, syrup, or infusion – everything you need to know about that is clearly defined in the beginning – before you even start learning about the powers of the herbs.

DEFINING HERBAL REMEDIES

At the very start of our journey together, let's explain what herbal medicine represents. Herbal medicine is, in fact, alternative medicine. Indeed, while today it is regarded as an alternative, in the past it was very much traditional. It has been used over the centuries to treat various ailments and is still used heavily in different parts of the world.

I remember, as a teen, being taken to a naturopathic doctor. At the time, I didn't understand why my parents would prioritize natural medicine. Shouldn't we just go to the doctor and get a prescription? Of course, I had no understanding of the effects of pharmaceuticals or why my parents would prefer a natural remedy wherever possible. As far as I was concerned, the pharmacy was where you went to get medications to cure everything. I had no idea then that there were natural alternatives!

Natural remedies became important to me when I went through a period of ill health that the doctors couldn't treat. Nothing major, I am thankful to say, but I was chronically sick. For about 2 years, I caught everything. I went to the doctor, I was given prescriptions but nothing worked. I felt terrible. In fact, I was sick so long, I forgot what it felt like to be healthy. At a friend's recommendation, I visited her naturopath and asked for help. And within about two months, I was feeling better and had an immune system that was beginning to work again. I was amazed that natural remedies could do much more than the pharmaceuticals I had relied on.

Now, I know that there is a place for medical doctors, and I still take medications when necessary. If I break a bone or need stitches, I go to the hospital. And you should do the same. If you have a condition that is controlled by medications, don't stop anything cold turkey! Your health and well-being are of the utmost importance. Always see and discuss your health with your medical practitioner. I think there is a good balance to be stuck between modern and herbal medicines. I see natural remedies as a way to promote my overall health and vitality.

In today's world, it has become increasingly common to use herbal remedies such as tea leaves, powdered versions, or herbal supplements to utilize their healing properties.

Know that herbal remedies can come from different parts of a plant. You may have to use the seeds of a certain plant or the leaves, the roots, the flowers, etc. It sounds like such an interesting approach to well-being! It all boils down to the condition you are dealing with. Different conditions require a different approach – and a different part of the plant!

The secret of each part of a plant lies in its properties. Every part of certain botanical plants comes with a unique set of properties, and when combined, they contribute to some incredible effects on the body.

However, herbal remedies are so much more than that. Other than being able to relieve pain, they can boost the natural processes of the body, and they can contribute to an improved and healthier self. Isn't that what we all want? The benefits are plenty – so much that I have dedicated an entire section under each plant to it!

So, for all of you who are new to the subject of alternative medicine, stay tuned! There is so much more to learn! From the history of herbal remedies to figuring out the best and most popular ones of today, this subject offers an incredible insight into a whole new aspect of taking care of your body. From matcha to ginger, you will discover a lot more than you hoped for!

WHY GO NATURAL?

There are more than just a few reasons to turn to herbal medicine. Choosing natural remedies will help you become the pillar of your family – wherever possible, keep them happy and healthy without the need to use pharmaceuticals. You don't even need to consult a health professional for minor ailments – relaxation teas and infusions to boost your overall health, juices you can make in the comfort of your kitchen – they are all healthy and a perfect addition to your dietary plan!

Another consideration is the cost savings. Making your own herbal recipes can be very cost-effective, in many cases using what you already have in your kitchen. Consulting with your health provider and incorporating some of the herbal remedies you will learn about in this book is the right approach. After all, safety comes first; before doing anything yourself, ensure it is a safe approach for you.

Of course, depending on the symptoms of your issue and your perspective, the approach may vary. But the bottom line is that if you have started reading this, you are eager to learn more about the incredible world of alternative medicine. I am all up for it and can't wait to help you get there! Before you start experimenting with all 158 of these herbal recipes, lets learn a little about the basic forms herbal remedies take and how to prepare them.

Finally, I want to invite you to join our Facebook community at

www.facebook.com/groups/homesteadmindset/

Be part of our Homestead Mindset Community where we can learn about herbs, gardening, stocking your pantry, and asking questions about homesteading.

It doesn't matter if you live in an apartment or have many acres. The mindset of being natural, returning to the land, being a little old-fashioned, being prepared, and providing for ourselves starts with how we think. Let's learn together!

A Gift Just For You

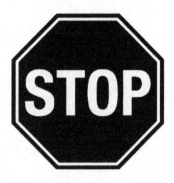

THANK YOU for purchasing my book. Because we share a love of healthy, wholesome, and natural living, I would love for you to have my very useful guide,

Build Your Own Natural First Aid Kit

- 11 Essential Herbal Remedies for Common Ailments
- 8 Important Natural Products
- 9 Necessary First Aid Tools to Be Prepared

To download your FREE GUIDE, scan this QR code

or go to
firstaid.homesteadmindset.com
If you need help, email me at hello@homesteadmindset.com

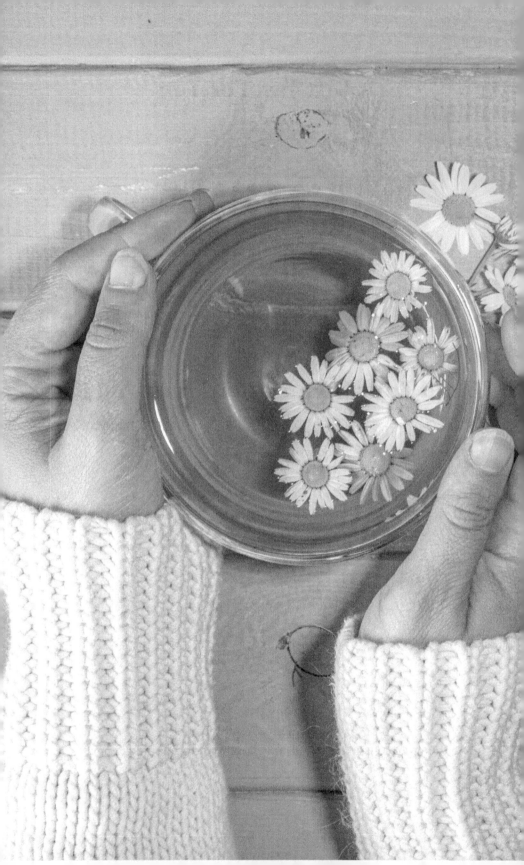

CHAPTER ONE

HOW TO MAKE NATURAL REMEDIES AT HOME

Making natural remedies from the comfort of your home has never been easier than it is today. Many people have gathered the knowledge and wisdom shared from generation to generation only to discover that there is a vast array of properties and uses for medicinal remedies. To make things even better, most of the recipes hardly require any cooking at all!

When you make an herbal remedy, it is essential to use the herb whose properties will help you heal. Moreover, the mixture will undergo a specific process (infusion, decoction, tincture, etc.), enabling you to extract the most potent benefits and help your body absorb or digest it properly. Herbal medicine has been used to support overall well-being – it is an excellent way to give yourself the chance to thrive!

TYPES OF HERBAL REMEDIES

Many people turn to herbal remedies as an additional form of nutrition because herbs are filled with vitamins and minerals beyond your imagination. They can support your gut health, your organs and systems, your hormones, your mood, and your sleep. Starting today, we will uncover the colorful world of herbal remedies.

The diverse range of remedies you will learn here will become the pillar of your holistic approach to health.

HOW TO MAKE YOUR OWN HERBAL REMEDY AT HOME

Before we start our journey into the multitude of herbal remedies, it's important that we define the commonly used terms for herbal remedies. In the book, when we refer to a "decoction" or a "tincture," please refer back to this chapter to review what it is and how to make each remedy. Believe me, soon you will have made each type of remedy so often this will become second nature. As the list is extensive, take a look at the numerous options before we go into details and recipes!

Below, there are also general recipes given as examples to those who are only getting started. You will learn how to make each base and add the herbs you like. The base is underlined everywhere, so you know exactly what you need to make it!

WATER EXTRACTS

A classic water extract is a tea. Soak the herb in hot water, like you would if making a tea, and then it is ready to drink. If properly used, water extracts can help you maintain your optimal health. Did you know that you can use a water extract to rinse your skin if you're sensitive to soap? And, of course, you can use it internally, too. Drink the flavored water you have made and enjoy.

That said, here are the basic steps to make any water extracts.

Ingredients:
- Filtered or distilled water
- Dried herbs

Supplies:
- Pot to boil (or anything in which you prefer making tea)
- Sterilized glass bottle with a lid or spray bottle in case it is for topical use
- Preservative (if it is to give it a longer shelf life)

Notes:

Using fresh herbs would introduce microbiological species, further complicating the preservation process, so make sure they are dry.

Using tap water is not recommended as it may contain bacteria.

The ratio should be 1:5 for herbs to water.

Make sure to boil the water and leave it for 5 minutes to cool off just a little bit, and then add the herbs. The water should not be left boiling with the herbs inside since this may cook them.

The water extract should be left for 30 minutes. If you are making a more potent extract, leave it overnight.

Inclure the herbs you neer anr make the water extract to your liking.

INFUSIONS

Infusions are slightly stronger than water extract. They are a natural and organic home product with medicinal value. Infusions can be used the same way as water extracts – drinking, bathing, cooking, and even making cosmetics.

Here are the basic steps to make any type of infusion.

Ingredients:
- A cup of hot water
- Dried herbs

Supplies:
- Pot to boil
- A jar or anything you can close tightly with a lid

Notes:
- You make an infusion by pouring boiling water over some dried herbs.
- Then, put the lid on so the non-aromatic volatile chemicals don't escape.
- Steep for 10-30 minutes, then strain.
- You should add 1 teaspoon per 1 boiled water cup or 1 tablespoon per 1 teapot.
- You can work with both fresh and dried herbs in this case.
- Infusions are best made with leaves, flowers, or even some fruit.

If you want to make an infusion at home, use any herb you need - or one that comes in handy!

DECOCTIONS

Decoctions require a little bit of simmering. So, when your water boils, and you add your herbs, the decoction is made by leaving it to simmer for at least 10 minutes. Slow cooking would work perfectly, so you may even want to use your crockpot for this. You should use a lid here to prevent it from boiling dry. Once your decoction is done simmering, you should strain it and store the liquid in an airtight jar to create a magnificent herbal remedy. You will get a nice syrupy concentrate with many uses and applications, as seen in some of our recipes.

Take a look at the decoction example recipe below - you can also use some sturdier ingredients such as woodier herbs and various herb parts. Consume daily.

Ingredients:
- ½ cup of the hard parts of dried herbs – seeds, roots, trunk bark, or mushrooms
- 1 liter of cold water

Supplies:
- A saucepan with a lid
- A large jar or flask to transfer and store the decoction

Notes:
- Add the ingredients into the saucepan and cover with a lid.
- Bring them to a boil, then turn down the heat and leave it to simmer for at least 30 minutes.
- Remove from heat and let it completely cool down.
- Strain the herbs and bottle the liquid. In a fridge, it can last up to 3-4 days.
- Once you have the decoction, you can strain the plant material out and reduce the liquid to a syrup consistency. In this form, it has similar powers to herbal extracts in pill forms you buy from the health store.

AROMATIC WATERS

Most of you have probably heard about rosewater – a fragrant liquid that does wonders for the body. It is an excellent herbal remedy to include in your home. The difference is in the making - when you make yours, you will notice small pools of essential oil floating on top.

Here is a recipe on how to make any refreshing aromatic water.

Ingredients:
- A generous amount of plant material
- Enough water to cover it

Supplies:
- A pan
- A heatproof bowl or a jug
- A heatproof ramekin
- Ice cubes

Notes:

- Place your herbs in the pan, and then add as much water as you need to cover them. Then turn on some gentle heat.
- Take the heat-proof ramekin and place it upside down on the bottom of the pan. On top, add the heat-proof bowl or jug. As a vessel, this should not collect water from the bottom as it is where the final product will be collected from.
- Place the pan lid upside down to create a path through which the water will drip from the lid into the heat-proof vessel.
- If you want to make the steam condense, place some ice cubes in the lid's bowl while ensuring none of them get inside.
- Due to strong potency, not all plants should be made this way. Research the herb before using it.
- Keep it in the fridge for as long as it stays fresh - about 6 months.

OIL EXTRACTS

From beeswax to cocoa butter, create oil extracts yourself and use them in foods as well as externally. When you prepare them, it is imperative to use a heatproof pan of gently simmering water and add as much oil as possible after placing your herb in it too. Then, you leave everything to simmer for at least three hours, and voila – make delightful preparations as easy as one, two, three!

If you need instant stress relief, you can make an oil extract at home and gently massage your temples with it.

Ingredients:
- A handful of any plant
- Enough oil to cover it
- Gently simmering water

Supplies:
- A heatproof glass bowl or a jug
- A pan
- A small bottle

14

Notes:
- Place the water in the pan and bring it to a boil, then down to a simmer.
- Add the heat-proof bowl or jug on top of it, place your herbs in it, and the oil.
- Three hours is the perfect time to leave this simmering on low heat, especially if you use fresh leaves and flowers.
- Dried herbs can be steeped in oil for days.
- It is important to keep the plant material submerged at all times, and once you're done, strain it through a fine sieve to keep even the smallest particles from getting through and spoiling it.

SYRUPS, HONEY, AND CANDIES

The common ground for all three of them includes creating a thick and gloopy mixture. They sweeten your day and preserve your health. The base mostly consists of dissolving sugar at a ratio of 2-parts sugar and 3-parts liquid. Then, add any aromatic herb you like. Once you create honey, candies, or sugar, they have vast uses – from cough candy to toppings for desserts.

Any herb you like will ₀o perfectly for the preparation of syrup.

Ingredients:
- 2 parts sugar
- 3 parts liquid
- A strong infusion or decoction

Supplies:
- A large pan
- Sterilized bottles

Notes:
- Bring the liquid and the sugar to a boil and then to a light simmer.
- Add the infusion and continue mixing until you get a thick, gloopy consistency.
- Transfer to sterilized bottles.

HERBAL VINEGAR

Homemade vinegar has multiple benefits, including antioxidant, anti-inflammatory, and anti-microbial properties. Sometimes, both cooking and drinks require a little bit of twist, and homemade herbal vinegar is the real deal. The easiest way is to add your herbs to a jar, fill the jar with vinegar, leave it tightly closed for a week, and enjoy. Make sure the vinegar completely covers the herbs, give it a shake or a stir daily, and then strain off the herbs and keep that delicious vinegar for future use.

When making your own herbal vinegar at home - the choice of herbs will ∢epen∢ on your nee∢s.

Ingredients:
- A bottle of vinegar
- Your choice of dried herb

Supplies:
- A sterilized jar
- A spray bottle to transfer your vinegar

Notes:
- Take your favorite herb and place it in the jar. Add the vinegar to completely fill up the jar (to the top) and close tightly with a lid.
- Leave it to macerate for up to a week.
- Transfer into small spray bottles and use.
- This vinegar can last up to a year if stored properly (in a cool and dark place).

ALCOHOL TINCTURES

If you want to expand your botanical remedy repertoire, you can use this alcohol tincture. It is a convenient homemade remedy and a great thing to utilize whenever you are suffering from indigestion or insomnia. You can use gin, brandy, wine, or vodka and macerate the herb for no more than 4 weeks to unlock its full potential.

Take a look at the base below, an• after making it, take the tincture orally by placing a few •rops of it un•er your tongue. Keep in min• that you can use any herb to prepare this.

Ingredients:
- Your choice of herbs
- An alcohol base (vodka, gin, brandy, wine)

Supplies:
- Jars with tight lids
- Bottles that close very well

Notes:
- Press down the herbs into the jar and cover that with the alcohol of your choosing.
- Seal the jars well, and shake them a few times a day for 14 days.
- Strain, but don't filter the liquid afterward.
- Add into bottles, close them tight, and keep in a cool and dry place.
- Shake well before use.
- A few drops mixed into some hot water will do the trick.

POULTICES

A poultice is something you use immediately after you notice a smaller skin injury you need to treat. Thankfully, it is so easy to make that you can do it in your kitchen and apply it to the affected area immediately.

Here is a base below – you can use any herb.

Ingredients:
- A handful of dried herbs
- A cup of water

Supplies:
- A small pan
- Cloth or gauze
- Cooking Oil (I prefer olive oil)

Notes:
- Boil the water and then bring it down to a simmer - add the herbs inside. Leave them for 2 minutes to simmer, then remove from heat.
- Rub the oil on the affected area to prevent the poultice from sticking. Then, take out the herb and apply it to the skin while it is still hot.
- Bandage the herb in place by using some gauze or a cloth. Leave it for up to 3 hours, and change if necessary.

CREAMS

Creams are similar to decoction and infusion since the process is almost the same. However, the uses vary, and with the creams, you will get a toxin-free and completely natural product that can help you nourish and hydrate and heal your skin.

You already know how to make a tincture, decoction, or infusion. Making the cream requires a few extra steps - see the recipe below. Keep in mind that you can make this with any herb!

Ingredients:
- 16 parts herb oil of your choosing
- 8 parts tincture, decoction, or infusion of your choice
- 4 parts good beeswax
- 4 parts vegetable oil or animal fat
- ¼ part powdered borax

Supplies:
- 2 double saucepans or bowls suspended over pots of boiling water
- Sterilized jars

Notes:
- Gently heat the beeswax and fat in one bowl and the herb oil in another one. Add the warm oil to the beeswax as soon as you notice it is fully melted.
- Heat the tincture and dissolve the borax powder in it. While continuously stirring, slowly add the borax solution to the beeswax and oil mix.
- Once everything is combined, remove it from the heat and stir to prevent it from separating.
- Pour the mixture into sterilized jars and use.

ESSENTIAL TOOLS EVERY HERBALIST NEEDS

As you may notice from the simple ways these types of herbal remedies are prepared, all the tools are likely already a part of your kitchen. However, all professional practitioners and beginners who are only dabbling in the subject know, there is a list of necessary essential tools when making herbal remedies. If you have them all handy – great, but if not, make sure they are always in a visible spot, within reach.

- *Cheesecloth* – this is your strainer and your best friend when creating your remedies
- *Pestle and mortar* – use them for fresh and dry herbs
- *Funnels* – get different sizes for different purposes
- *Double boiler insert* – make your transfer trouble-free while melting down the wax and herbal oils
- *Sprouting screen* – it is a convenient way to create your favorite herbal infusions
- *Jars* – this one is a given, jars with lids that seal, are a must
- *Kitchen scale* – use it to measure the amount of the ingredients whenever you decide to create an herbal remedy
- *Tea press and strainer* – keep both of them handy as you never know when you might want to enjoy a homemade brew
- *Sterilize bottles and spray bottles* – Sterilizing all your storage bottles is the key to longevity for any of your creations.

SAFETY PRECAUTIONS YOU NEED TO TAKE WHEN USING HERBAL REMEDIES

Herbs and the entire practice of herbal medicine can be incredibly useful. You can take care of many health concerns with the help of a mixture, or a specific herb. Now, as you reviewed the benefits, a thought may have crossed your mind – what precautions do I need to know about?

As with every powerful thing, you need to be aware when using herbal remedies. Being used for a long time ensures that it is typically a safe practice, but, everybody is different. Your body might be more prone to or resistant to some of the properties, so approach new usage with caution at first. Here are a few safety precautions to keep in mind:

Herbs are not pharmaceutical drugs – they work differently from traditional medications, meaning the approach you must take will differ. The method includes discovering the main concern of your issue rather than looking to overcome any issue with drugs only. Herbal medicine enhances an approach where you look within, with a holistic method, and try to support the natural healing mechanisms of the body.

On many occasions, herbs are what you can use to enhance the production of anything the body needs and create the perfect balance. Then, you can reap the benefits.

Listen to your body – the body speaks with actions. Whenever an herb does the body well, it manifests good signs. You have elevated levels of energy, your sleep schedule is better, and you don't experience any pain.

But, if you start noticing some issues with your body after taking an herbal remedy, that means it does not sit well with your body. In this case, the most common signals of the body include a bloated stomach, an upset stomach, and an overall feeling of being unwell.

Ultimately, we must face that not all herbs are for everybody. One of the first things you need to do is listen to your body and fulfill its wishes.

Start small – you don't need to try all herbs at once. Make a schedule of what you want to try, and with the help of a professional – when to try it. Start with the gentlest herbs and smaller doses. Gradually build your way up and reach the most intense ones! As you move forward, you can even increase the dose too.

Also, consider how severe your condition is. Some conditions require immediate attention and a high dosage of a powerful herb. This is a quicker treatment. If you are uncertain of where to begin, check with a professional – they can give you some guidance in the right direction.

Taking medications – if you are already taking medication, it is best to talk to your healthcare provider and a holistic professional, too, to determine the next steps. Some individuals take medication and turn to herbal remedies at the same time. The danger is there could be many contradictions. Err on the side of caution and always consult your health professional.

Some of the interactions that can hurt the body include mixing blood-thinning drugs with almost any herbs and pain medications with sedative herbs. Also, if you use detox herbs, they can clear out the medication from your system before they've had the chance to work on you.

Opt for combining herbs and medication that cannot counteract each other. Avoid a combination that can be problematic and turn to combine herbs that can interact with each other instead.

Advocate for yourself – do proper research before starting herbal medicine. There is extensive research to be done on the subject, so start as early as today. Reach out to a few professionals in the field and pick their brains on the subject. You can easily find some credible sources and turn to one to be your constant assistant.

As long as it is your health in question, you need to advocate for yourself. Talk to them frequently about dosages and look for established herbalist resources to back up any claims you might have. Herbalists can help you understand how a certain herb functions on a deeper level. Time frames and isolated components – ask all the important questions!

Herbal medicine is one of the safest forms you will ever find. The herbs used in the past are still being used today. You can practice herbal medicine effectively and safely – all you need to do is try. And please don't forget that while this book will teach you many wonderful new remedies, it cannot diagnose your concerns or know your pre-existing conditions. So always consult a health professional with any questions.

After you have gone through some of the simple basic steps and information about how to begin preparing the most widespread herbal remedies, I hope you are excited to get to work! Let's start uncovering the secret recipes and ingredients and learn new information about frequently used herbs that will give you wonderful health advantages.! We will start by learning about the digestive system and how to balance your gut health – an important challenge many people try to tackle. The next chapter is all about alternative remedies for digestive health.

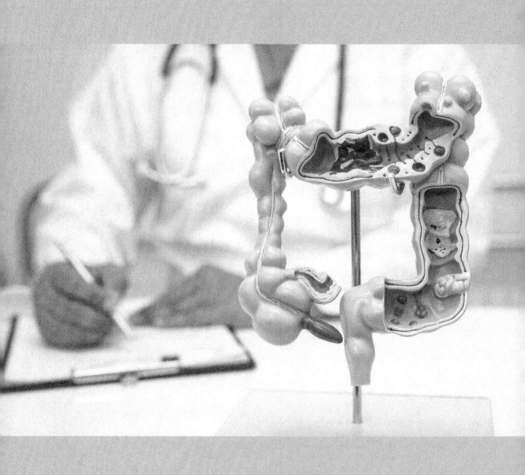

CHAPTER TWO

REMEDIES FOR DIGESTIVE (GUT) HEALTH

There is no worse feeling in the world than having to deal with unhealthy gut issues. It is a breeding ground for various ailments and can contribute to some serious long-term health issues. Have you ever wondered how that comes to be?

As people grow, they tend to develop various habits and adopt a certain lifestyle. In most cases, they try to be on the safer side, implementing some healthy habits that will keep them happy and energized. But when life and responsibilities hit, the changing patterns can affect the overall way of living, including what foods you consume.

This can, in turn, lead to some serious gut issues. Consuming larger amounts of highly processed foods can contribute to becoming lactose intolerant, experiencing leaky gut syndrome, and many other conditions. On top of that, many physical and mental issues can further develop from an unhealthy gut. The stomach is one of the parts of the body that needs the most attention since a dysfunctional gut can contribute to an overall decrease in the quality of life.

This chapter is all about maintaining a functional and healthy gut. Balance is always needed, and now you get the chance to learn how to do it yourself

– from the comfort of your home. Discover healthy homemade recipes for a healthy gut.

WHAT IS A HEALTHY GUT?

A healthy gut functions well, contains a balanced and diverse microbiome, results in optimal digestion and nutrient absorption, and minimizes discomfort and pain. The gut comprises large and small intestines, plays an important role in the overall body's health, and is the sole organ responsible for processing and taking in nutrients from everything you consume. This process supports the immune system and creates a barrier that keeps you safe from harmful substances.

HERBAL REMEDIES FOR BALANCING YOUR GUT HEALTH

Finding the right concoction to help you balance your gut health can be a lengthy process – if you do it alone. The ingredients below can help you discover a wide range of remedies you can do yourself – both easy to make and easy on the body. Let's see what you can make!

1. GINGER TEA (ZINGIBER OFFICINALE)

 Medicinal Properties – Some of the best medicinal properties of ginger tea are helpful with chronic gut inflammation. Consuming it will help you debloat, handle any pain or constipation, and help with IBS, IDS, and other conditions.

If you add some lemon and honey to it, you will get an even more delicious drink that you may want to drink – just for the pleasure of it.

Fun Fact – ginger is not actually a root – it is a rhizome, an underground plant stem.

 Why Will It Help – because it has both a soothing and an invigorating power.

 How to Make It

Ingredients – 2cm (0.8 inch) fresh ginger, a cup of water, ½ lemon, and a teaspoon of honey.

Instructions – Wash and slice the lemon. Grate your ginger, then add them to a tea strainer, along with the hot cup of water. Leave it for about two minutes (check the first chapter under infusions).

 How to Use It – consume it whenever you want to experience gut relief – about 500ml (2 cups) daily.

2. DIGESTIVE TEA

 Medicinal Properties – This is a mixture of several powerful herbs that will promote good health and soothe your upset stomach. It promotes gut health, especially in cases when you often feel gassy and experience diarrhea, constipation, and bloating.

 Fun Fact – Peppermint can relax the muscles, lemon balm eases discomfort, and fenugreek is filled with antioxidants and fiber!

 Why Will It Help – Not only are these ingredients packed with antioxidants and polyphenols, but they also have specific compounds with the ability to soothe, heal, and help your digestive enzymes.

 How to Make It

Ingredients – 1 teaspoon dried peppermint, 1 teaspoon dried lemon balm, 1 teaspoon fenugreek, 1 lemon (cut in slices), 1 stick of cinnamon, and some water.

Instructions – Combine the peppermint, fenugreek, and lemon balm in a pot and add the water. Bring them to a boil and remove from heat. Add the fresh lemon slices and the cinnamon stick and steep for about 10 minutes. Strain – it is ready to use (check the first chapter, under infusions).

 How to Use It – simply pour it into a mug and enjoy it. Always sip on it while you are having a meal. Best served warm.

3. PEPPERMINT, LICORICE, AND NETTLE TEA (MENTHA PIPERITA, GLYCYRRHIZA GLABRA & URTICA)

 Medicinal Properties – Peppermint tea is excellent for gas, bloating, and upset stomach. Licorice is not only a promoter of healthy digestion but also calms the nervous system down. Finally, the nettle is filled with magnesium, helping relax the muscles and detox the body.

 Fun Fact – Licorice is also known for treating respiratory tract issues and several skin conditions.

 Why Will It Help – When combined, these three ingredients can help along the entire digestive process. Peppermint has high magnesium levels, soothing the nervous system and colon muscles; the nettle brings on board minerals that help detoxify your body, and licorice lowers any indigestion symptoms.

 How to Make It
Ingredients – 2 tablespoons loose peppermint leaves, 1 tablespoon loose licorice tea leaves, 2 tablespoons loose nettle tea leaves, 4 cups of water.

Instructions – You can use both dried and fresh leaves. Boil the water and then pour it over the ingredients in a pot. Steep for 10 minutes, strain, and serve (check the first chapter under infusions).

How to Use It – Drink this delicious digestion tea in the evening and let your body relax.

4. GUT-HEALING TEA

Medicinal Properties – The compounds from this gut-healing tea act as effective remedies for conditions where the gut is damaged, inflamed, or irritated. It is composed of several herbs, including roses, marshmallow root, and cinnamon.

Fun Fact – In medieval times, roses were often associated with sacrifice and were used to decorate the tombs of martyrs. After that, they were a symbol of luxury and religious devotion.

Why Will It Help – If you are looking for a tea that will focus on the digestive tract, reducing inflammation, damage, and irritation, you should try this one.

How to Make It
Ingredients – 2 teaspoons marshmallow root, 2 teaspoons dried plantain (*Plantago major*) leaf, 1 teaspoon cinnamon chips or 2 cinnamon sticks, 1 teaspoon rose petals, 6 cloves, 2-star anise pods (whole or crushed), 1 liter of water.

Instructions – Prepare it as a basic decoction or a weaker infusion, and let it steep for at least 60 minutes in an insulated thermos (check the first chapter, under infusions and decoctions).

How to Use It – Drink this tea regularly (the minimum is a quart each day) and support healthy and gentle detoxification.

5. HOMEMADE DIGESTION LOZENGES

 Medicinal Properties – the powerful properties of the ingredients will boost digestion and will help you feel better. This is due to the cardamom, which can alleviate gas and bloating; ginger – which helps immensely with moving the food throughout the whole digestive system; licorice root – which will soothe any acid reflux and heartburn, and, of course, acacia powder, which acts as a prebiotic. Prebiotics are the food for probiotics to grow and nourish the digestive system.

 Fun Fact – Cardamom is one of the most exotic spices in the world (and one of the oldest, too).

 Why Will It Help – because it will soothe the feeling of being overly full and bloated and will ease discomfort.

 How to Make It
Ingredients – 4 parts organic maple or coconut sugar, 2 parts cardamom powder, 1 part ginger root powder, 1 part licorice root powder, 1 part acacia powder, and some distilled water.

Instructions – Combine the herbs with the sugar in a bowl. Add a drop of distilled water with a dropper, incorporating it as you go. Do this until you create a consistency of cookie dough. Form into small lozenges. Let them dry on a plate for a few days, and store them in a glass jar.

 How to Use It – take one after dinner as a digestif.

HERBAL REMEDIES TO HELP WITH IBS (IRRITABLE BOWEL SYNDROME)

The name of this condition says it all – it can irritate you! Other than regular medication, turn to some herbal remedies that can provide instant relief.

6. ALOE VERA SMOOTHIE (ALOE BARBADENSIS MILLER)

 Medicinal Properties – This superfood contains a large amount of water, 20 minerals, 12 vitamins, and 200 active plant compounds (also called phytonutrients), making it an impressive addition to your kitchen.

 Fun Fact – aloe vera has a similar flavor to the cucumber.

Why Will It Help – Because of the soothing effects, it can relieve cramping, flatulence, bloating, and abdominal pain – all symptoms of IBS.

 How to Make It

Ingredients – 1 cup of almond or coconut milk, 1 medium-sized aloe vera leaf, ½ cup fresh or frozen blueberries, ½ cup fresh or frozen mango pieces, ½ tablespoon coconut oil, 1 handful fresh basil, some honey to taste.

Instructions – Put all the ingredients into a blender and blend it until smooth.

 How to Use It – drink up!

7. TRIPHALA TEA (EMBLICA OFFICINALIS)

 Medicinal Properties – packed with antioxidant, antibacterial, antiviral, antispasmodic, and antifungal properties, it can heal the symptoms of IBS.

 Fun Fact – The Triphala tea has been a pillar of Ayurvedic medicine for a long time just because of its digestive properties.

Why Will It Help – Even though it is generally used as a body tonic, it can cleanse and detox the system and deal with bloating, abdominal pain, constipation, and indigestion.

 How to Make It
Ingredients – ½ teaspoon triphala powder, 250ml (1 cup) of water, 1 cinnamon stick.

Instructions – Add the powder to the pot along with the water. Bring it to a boil. Then add the cinnamon and let it simmer for 10 minutes, or longer to get a more powerful cinnamon flavor. Remove from heat and pour in a cup.

 How to Use It – Consume the tea as soon as you prepare it.

8. GOLDEN MILK TURMERIC TEA (CURCUMA LONGA)

 Medicinal Properties – They include reducing arthritis pain, joint pain, and inflammation, as a cure for depression, and last but not least – doing wonders for the digestive tract.

 Fun Fact – India is the largest turmeric producer, and before naming it turmeric, it was called Indian Saffron.

 Why Will It Help – The antioxidant and anti-inflammatory properties of golden milk make it not only the perfect evening ritual addition but can also help soothe your digestive system.

 How to Make It
Ingredients – 1 cup organic unsweetened nut milk or coconut milk, ½ teaspoon ground turmeric, a pinch of black pepper, 1 small piece of ginger root (grated and peeled), 1 big pinch of ground cinnamon, 1 big pinch of ground cardamom, and ¼ teaspoon raw honey.

Instructions – Put all the ingredients in a bowl and whisk them together. Then, place them on the stove over medium heat for 15 minutes. Allow it to simmer, but not boil.

 How to Use It – drink a cup any time of the day (though preferably in the evening).

9. ARTICHOKE LEAF TINCTURE (CYNARA CARDUNCULUS)

 Medicinal Properties – The artichoke leaf contains antioxidants and probiotics, supporting digestion, healthy blood lipids, and detoxification.

 Fun Fact – Although the artichoke is often considered a vegetable, it is actually a type of thistle.

 Why Will It Help – The bitter taste is not a favorite to the taste buds, but it will ease digestive discomfort and promote strong and healthy digestion, diminishing the symptoms of IBS.

 How to Make It
Ingredients – 1 ounce dried artichoke leaf, 5 ounces of 60-80 proof of alcohol.

Instructions – Add the artichoke to a jar and pour the alcohol over it. Close the jar and shake well. Place it in a dark and cool area, and shake the jar occasionally. When it is ready, squeeze the mixture through a cheesecloth, pour the liquid into a sterilized bottle, and use (refer to the first chapter, under alcohol tinctures)

 How to Use It – Consume a few drops, distilled with water.

10. PSYLLIUM SEED HUSK (PLANTAGO OVATA)

 Medicinal Properties – These seeds are an ancient treatment for IBS because of their high soluble fiber content. They can clean the colon and improve overall digestive tract function.

 Fun Fact – It can both form your stool and soften stool. It is also a great alternative to eggs when baking!

 Why Will It Help – you will gain much more than you bargained for. Because of its powers, it can help deal with your IBS symptoms, abdominal pain, nausea or vomiting, constipation, flatulence, abdominal cramping, appendicitis, and gastritis.

 How to Make It
Ingredients – 1 teaspoon of seeds in 240ml (about 1 cup) of water.
Instructions – Mix the ingredients and drink up.

 How to Use It – The recommended course of action is to drink plenty of liquid while consuming it.

HERBAL TREATMENTS FOR HELICOBACTER PYLORI

Even though it is one of the most common bacteria found in up to 70% of the world's population, if not treated on time, it can cause many discomforts and serious conditions. These include nausea and vomiting, blood in stool, diarrhea, bloating, loss of appetite, and weight loss, along with burning gut pain and frequent burping. However, it can also lead to ulcers, ulcerative colitis, and many serious chronic illnesses.

To significantly reduce Helicobacter pylori in the digestive tract, you should find the most beneficial herbal remedy. From the list below, you can discover the most popular recipes – try one (or a few) and stick with the one that works best for you.

11. CRANBERRY JUICE (VACCINIUM OXYCOCCOS)

 Medicinal Properties – Since cranberries come with many Medicinal Properties , the best include reducing inflammation within the body and helping with digestive issues.

 Fun Fact – Cranberries are also excellent for your teeth because they keep the bacteria from sticking on them. This additionally prevents H.pylory from entering through the root canal into the body.

 Why Will It Help – Even though consumption of cranberry juice has increased due to its delicious flavor, it will not only aid the Helicobacter pylori in its first stage, but it will preserve the natural gut microbe.

 How to Make It
Ingredients – 2 quarts of water, 8 cups of fresh or frozen cranberries, ½ cup of sugar, ½ cup of lemon juice, ½ cup of orange juice.

Instructions – Put the cranberries in a pot, add the water, and bring them to a boil. Then reduce the heat and leave them to simmer for about 20 minutes until the berries start popping. Remove from heat, strain the mixture, discard the berries, and return the liquid to the pot. Add the other ingredients, return the pot to the heat, and bring to a boil – stir until the sugar fully dissolves. Remove from heat, cool off, and transfer to a pitcher.

 How to Use It – Drink at least 250ml (1 cup) of cranberry juice a day to see positive results.

12. LEMONGRASS OIL IN AROMATHERAPY (CYMBOPOGON)

 Medicinal Properties – Having the power to treat insomnia and restlessness makes lemongrass a powerful addition to your first aid kit. In addition, its sedative effect will soothe any Helicobacter Pylori-induced pain.

 Fun Fact – Lemongrass is an excellent source of magnesium, zinc, and iron.

 Why Will It Help – Because lemongrass comes with a mild sedative effect, it can help ease your discomfort and pain.

 How to Make It
Ingredients – A few drops of lemongrass oil and some water.

Instructions – Fill the diffuser with water and add a few drops of the lemongrass essential oil.

 How to Use It – use it whenever necessary.

13. GREEN TEA (CAMELLIA SINENSIS)

 Medicinal Properties – Contains antioxidant polyphenols and caffeine, an amazing combo that fights off H. Pylori.

 Fun Fact – Green tea contains no calories at all.

 Why Will It Help – In terms of H. Pylori infections, it can reduce the side effects that are created by the antibiotics that treat this condition.

How to Make It

Ingredients – 1 teaspoon of green tea and a cup of hot water.

Instructions – Add the green tea to the cup and let that steep for about 5-10 minutes. Then strain and transfer to a cup.

How to Use It – Consume this tea daily (up to two times a day) to reap the benefits.

14. ALOE VERA JUICE (ALOE BARBADENSIS MILLER)

Medicinal Properties – Aloe vera contains anti-inflammatory compounds and can alleviate pain all over the body, both inside and out.

Fun Fact – There are about 250 species of aloe vera in the world, but only 4 of them are cultivated for their health benefits to humans.

Why Will It Help – It contains antimicrobial effects that can fight off H. Pylori, and it works great as an adjuvant therapy when combined with other antibiotics.

How to Make It

Ingredients – 1 aloe vera leaf, 1 cup of water, and any type of juice (optional).

Instructions – Scrape the gel out of the aloe vera leaf and put it inside a blender. Add the water and blend until smooth. If you want, you can add the juice of your choice to add some flavor. Blend again.

How to Use It – Put the juice in a cup and drink it up! You can drink this juice once or every alternate day for a couple of weeks.

15. BLACK CUMIN SEEDS AND HONEY MIXTURE (NIGELLA SATIVA & MEL)

 Medicinal Properties – The overall Medicinal Properties include antioxidant, and anti-inflammatory properties, and the ability to boost your entire immunity and maintain the health of your heart.

 Fun Fact – The therapeutic properties of the black cumin seeds protect the body from chronic diseases and cell damage.

 Why Will It Help – When combined, these two create a powerful combo that provides the body with anti-dyspeptic effects (these include burning in the gut, bloating, nausea that happens after eating, etc.), ultimately easing and possibly eradicating the H. Pylori infection.

 How to Make It
Ingredients – 1 teaspoon of ground black cumin seeds and 2 teaspoons of raw honey.

Instructions – Mix a teaspoon of the ground black cumin seeds with the honey until they create a homogenous paste.

 How to Use It – Consume this mixture once a day until you notice that your symptoms are improving.

HERBAL REMEDIES FOR STOMACH ULCERS AND GASTRITIS

If you are dealing with a horrible case of gastritis or stomach ulcers, try a remedy beyond the powers of regular medicine. Instead of dealing with antibiotics for a long time, consider turning to natural remedies that will promote healing more effectively and naturally.

16. INDIAN GOOSEBERRY JUICE (PHYLLANTHUS EMBLICA)

 Medicinal Properties – The immune-boosting properties of Indian gooseberries make this a vibrant addition to your lifestyle. Even though they are sour to taste, that has not stopped people from reaping their benefits. They are rich in Vitamins C, A, and E, and have antioxidant properties that improve overall digestive health.

 Fun Fact – Gooseberries are smaller than a plum but larger than a grape.

 Why Will It Help – No matter how you decide to consume them, they can help your body deal with the effects of gastric ulcers.

 How to Make It
Ingredients – ½ cup plain water, coconut water, or any type of fruit juice, 6 Indian gooseberries (chopped), ½ inch peeled and chopped ginger.

Instructions – For this recipe, it is best to use fresh berries. Place all the ingredients in a blender/grinder and blend/grind until you get a smooth paste. Strain this to a pitcher using a spoon that will help you press out all the liquid from it.

 How to Use It – Consume the juice immediately. You can store it in the fridge for up to two days, but it might lose some of its nutrients.

17. KATUKI POWDER AND SUGAR (PICRORHIZA KURROOA)

 Medicinal Properties – From kidney health to liver health and, of course, digestive support – there is nothing this bitter root can't do! It acts as a potent detoxifier, anti-inflammatory, and antibiotic agent.

Fun Fact – Katuki helps remove the excessive heat from the body.

 Why Will It Help – The many benefits that come from the katuki can decrease inflammation and potentially heal an ulcer. This is very beneficial with acid peptic disorders.

 How to Make It
Ingredients – 2 grams of katuki powder, sugar to taste.
Instructions – Mix the ingredients until they are fully combined.

 How to Use It – Consume this mixture twice daily after a meal.

18. DOOB GRASS MIXTURE (CYNODON DACTYLON)

 Medicinal Properties – It contains unique properties that are excellent for dealing with stomach-related issues. It can detox the body and is filled with calcium, sodium, potassium, flavonoids, phosphorus, carbohydrates, and proteins.

 Fun Fact – The origin of doob (or durva) grass is the savannas of Africa.

 Why Will It Help – Other than treating a fever, it can help deal with an ulcer, a stomach infection, and other health issues. It contains antimicrobial and antiviral properties.

 How to Make It
Ingredients – 3-4 tablespoons of doob grass juice, a glass of water.

Instructions – If you only have fresh doob grass, then make the juice from it first. You can do this by using a mixer grinder – put 1 cup of doob grass and ½ cup of water. Use a cotton cloth to filter it through. Store it in the fridge and consume only 3-4 tablespoons of the juice dissolved in water. If you have dry doob grass, you can prepare tea using 1-2 teaspoons and hot water (but not boiling). Let it release its properties into the hot water for 10 minutes, and then strain and drink it.

 How to Use It – Drink for 15-30 days every morning on an empty stomach.

Keeping your body healthy and happy on the inside is just as important as keeping it healthy and happy on the outside. Discovering the wondrous and versatile benefits of herbal remedies and the powerful ingredients that will maintain gut health is a pleasure in itself.

But some of you might be eager to get to the next bit – skin health. There is much to cover on that front, so jump into the subject on the next page!

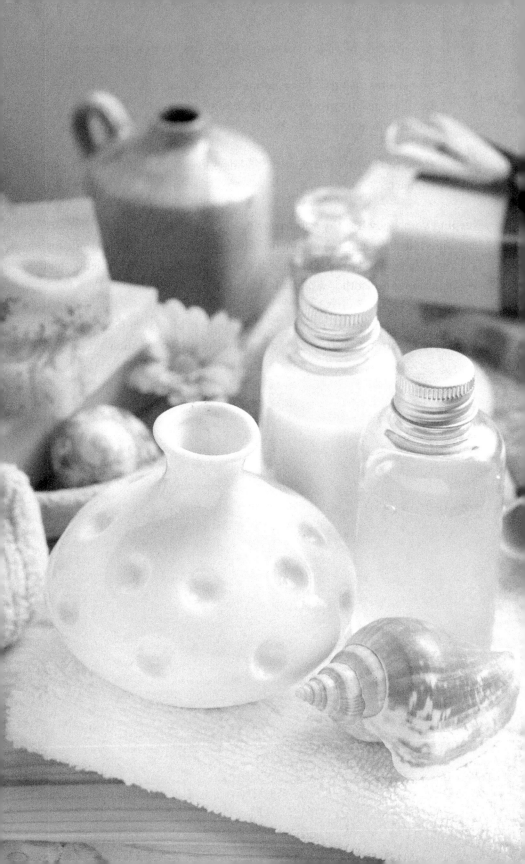

CHAPTER 3

REMEDIES FOR SKIN HEALTH

Health is what we give our bodies, which shows through our skin.

When you think about skin, what is the first thing that comes to mind? Is clear skin the first thing you thought of? Or maybe a problematic one? Your skin's appearance often reflects how well you care for your body.

Also, let's be honest – having a lot of skin imperfections can lead to lowered self-esteem and many other issues. I remember, as a teen, having the typical acne problem and feeling so self-conscious. And I just spoke to a friend yesterday who is very upset by the rosia she is experiencing. My daughters spent a lot of time filtering and editing their selfies before they deemed them ready to appear on social media!

Today, although the skincare world is highly developed and marketed, there are some ingredients that irritate some people's skin or contain chemicals that should be avoided. And there are some wonderful organic alternatives to consider. If your skin is more sensitive and/or susceptible to breakouts, natural ingredients may be your only choice. If your goal is simply to look your best and keep your skin in its beautiful glowing state, how much better to do it naturally and at a fraction of the cost? And who wants to expose your skin to unnecessary chemicals when natural home remedies can do the same things and perhaps even better?

Rather than delving into the subject of harmful and helpful compounds, why not go fully natural? Alternative medicine has always been much more than that – it can provide you with fantastic skincare options at home. Some herbs are so effective that they can make your skin glow!

Whether you are dealing with a skin issue or simply want to take extra care of yourself, there are many herbal options to try – see for yourself.

HERBAL REMEDIES FOR ACNE:

See some of the best herbal remedies that can help you treat acne in no time below.

19. ASHOKA PASTE (SARACA ASOCA)

 Medicinal Properties – Many essential nutrients are found in the Ashoka, including calcium, iron, essential oils, glycoside, tannins, and ketosterol.

 Fun Fact – The Ashoka tree bark is beneficial for treating menstrual issues such as uterine problems and abdominal pain.

 Why Will It Help – Because it has the power to remove toxins from the blood, making it super beneficial for the health of the skin (and overall acne prevention).

 How to Make It
Ingredients – Get 1 teaspoon of Ashoka powder and 0.5 oz of water.
Instructions – Mix until you create a thick paste.

 How to Use It – Apply the solution directly onto the acne and leave it for 3-5 minutes.

20. FLAX SEED POWDER OR OIL (LINUM USITATISSIMUM)

 Medicinal Properties – The healing properties of the flax seeds come from their high essential fatty acid content. They play an important role in keeping the sebum production normal.

 Fun Fact – Flaxseed oil is often taken in the form of a capsule!

 Why Will It Help – Because it is known as one of the best healing foods for acne, keeping the production of androgens under control and preventing acne.

 How to Make It
Ingredients - 1-2 tablespoons of flaxseeds, 2 cups of water, 1-2 tablespoons of oil.

Instruction - Start by boiling the water and then bring it down to a simmer. Use Chapter One to continue making this under oil extracts.

 How to Use It – consume two tablespoons orally daily.

21. CAMPHOR OIL (CINNAMOMUM CAMPHORA)

 Medicinal Properties – Camphor oil provides the skin with anti-inflammatory and soothing properties, giving some amazing benefits to the skin, including minimizing the appearance of acne.

 Fun Fact – You can also use camphor for skin whitening!

 Why Will It Help – Because it can relieve itching and inflammation due to its antibacterial and antifungal properties.

 How to Make It

Ingredients - 2 tablespoons ground camphor, 2 cups of water, 1-2 tablespoons of oil.

Instruction - Begin just like with the flaxseed oil, start by boiling the water and then bring it down to a simmer. Use Chapter One to make this at home, under oil extracts.

 How to Use It – Once you prepare the camphor oil, dilute a few drops of it in water and apply with a cotton pad to the skin every day to the affected area, until the acne is gone.

HERBAL REMEDIES FOR ROSACEA

Known as a long-term inflammatory skin condition, rosacea can happen to anyone. Learn how to deal with it naturally and safely from the comfort of your kitchen.

22. ORCHID TREE LEAF EXTRACT (BAUHINIA VARIEGATA)

 Medicinal Properties – Everything that the orchid contains is beneficial for the skin – zinc, magnesium, and calcium.

 Fun Fact – Did you know that the vanilla bean comes from a species of Orchid?

 Why Will It Help – Because it will not only calm down the irritation and soothe the skin but will also boost skin immunity and reduce the signs of aging and fine lines.

 How to Make It
Ingredients - 2 teaspoons of orchid tree leaf, 2 cups of water, 1-2 tablespoons of oil.

Instruction - Start by boiling the water and then bring it down to a simmer. Use Chapter One to make this at home, under oil extracts.

 How to Use It – gently apply it to the affected area with a cotton ball daily.

23. CANNABIS SEED OIL (CANNABIS SATIVA)

 Medicinal Properties – Cannabis has proven extremely helpful in overall skin health – from dealing with inflammation and supporting the skin barrier to minimizing breakouts.

 Fun Fact – It is extremely sustainable and planet-friendly, it is perfect for all skin types, and it will not get you high.

 Why Will It Help – Because it is filled with antioxidants, vitamins, and fatty acids, it can visibly reduce the redness caused by rosacea.

 How to Make It
Ingredients - 1-ounce cannabis buds/leaves, 2 cups of water, 2 cups of oil.

Instruction - Start by grinding the buds. If you have leaves, continue by spreading them on some baking paper and put them in your oven. Bake them for 60 minutes (after preheating your oven to 225 F). Then continue making this using Chapter One, under oil extracts.

 How to Use It – Apply a few drops of the oil to the affected areas and rub gently in a small circular motion.

HERBAL REMEDIES FOR ECZEMA

The condition known for causing itchy, dry, and inflamed skin is more common in children than in any other age group. Instead of having to deal with eczema's symptoms daily, here is how to treat it yourself.

24. COMMON PURSLANE LEAVES CONCOCTION (PORTULACA OLERACEA)

 Medicinal Properties – It contains antioxidants, vitamins, and omega-3 fats.

 Fun Fact – In addition to treating eczema, purslane will provide your skin with elasticity and reduce wrinkles.

 Why Will It Help – Because it is not only an adventurous choice, it is a healthy one too! It contains anti-inflammatory and antioxidant properties.

 How to Make It
Ingredients - 1 tablespoon of dried purslane leaves mixed with water.

Instructions - Bring the water to a boil and let it cool down for a bit. Check the first chapter – under water extracts to continue.

 How to Use It – consume daily. Consult with a healthcare professional to determine the proper dose for you.

25. OATS EXTRACT (AVENA SATIVA)

 Medicinal Properties – It works as an exfoliant, helping remove all the dead skin cells and oil and dirt buildup. Also, it reduces inflammation and moistures the skin.

Fun Fact – Using oat extract will also improve your skin tone, lighten it, and smooth out the texture.

 Why Will It Help – This is a very popular home remedy, and many people use it for dry and irritated skin. This home remedy can do wonders for anyone dealing with eczema.

 How to Make It
Ingredients - 1 ½ cups rolled oats, 2 cups of water, 2 tablespoons of carrier oil.

Instruction - Make the decoction or infusion with the rolled oats and continue the recipe as explained in Chapter 1 under creams.

 How to Use It – Apply to the affected areas daily.

26. QING DAI EXTRACT (INDIGO NATURALIS)

 Medicinal Properties – It is anti-inflammatory and promotes eczema and psoriasis-free skin.

 Fun Fact – Qing means clean or pure, referring to how extremely beneficial this herb is.

 Why Will It Help – Because it is anti-inflammatory and effective in soothing redness and itchiness when it comes to various skin conditions, including eczema.

 How to Make It
Ingredients - 1-2 teaspoons of Qing dai powder, 2 cups of water, 1-2 tablespoons of oil.

Instruction - Bring the water to a boil. Then proceed to make the oil extract by using the recipe guidelines in Chapter One.

How to Use It – Apply topically to the infected area.

27. NEEM OIL (AZADIRACHTA INDICA)

 Medicinal Properties – Neem oil contains anti-inflammatory and antibacterial properties, and one of its most famous treatments is for acne. However, using it regularly on your skin will soothe the inflamed areas caused by eczema.

 Fun Fact – Rubbing neem oil on your skin can keep mosquitos away during the summer months.

 Why Will It Help – It will help diminish the itchiness and redness, and since you can use it for acne, too, it can prevent future outbreaks.

 How to Make It
Ingredients - 1-2 teaspoons ground neem leaves, enough oil to cover it, 2-3 cups of water.

Instruction - Begin by bringing the water to a boil and then proceed to make the oil yourself using the guidelines from Chapter One, under oil extracts.

 How to Use It – Lightly dab the oil onto the affected areas with a cotton ball, leave it for about 20 minutes, and wash off the oil with lukewarm water.

DERMATITIS

A common skin irritation that can happen to anyone. It sometimes makes the skin crust and flake off, blister, and ooze. Here are a few ways you can deal with that.

28. OREGON GRAPE (MAHONIA AQUIFOLIUM)

 Medicinal Properties – Due to its anti-inflammatory and antimicrobial properties, it has become a popular ingredient for both topical and oral use, often found in tinctures, creams, and oil extracts.

 Fun Fact – The Oregon grape does not produce grapes.

 Why Will It Help – Dermatitis is an inflammatory skin condition, and the Oregon grape can deal with it because of its anti-inflammatory, anti-microbial, anti-fungal, and anti-bacterial properties, along with eczema.

 How to Make It

Ingredients - ½ cup of Oregon grape root (ground), 1 liter of cold water (for the decoction), and 16 parts herb oil, 4 parts beeswax, 4 parts vegetable oil, and ¼ part of powdered borax.

Instruction - Once you make your decoction, use Chapter One to create your Oregon grape cream.

 How to Use It – Apply topically every day for at least a month.

29. GINKGO BILOBA TABLETS (GINKGO BILOBA)

 Medicinal Properties – Ginkgo Biloba is best known for treating memory issues, but it also has properties that are treating other conditions, including skin issues. It is filled with antioxidants, protecting the skin from the damage done by free radicals. It also contains antibacterial properties.

 Fun Fact – It is one of the oldest living tree species in the world.

Why Will It Help – Because it is an anti-inflammatory elixir that will ease your dermatitis fast. It will increase moisture retention in the skin and reduce roughness.

 How to Make It
Ingredients - 1.76 oz ginkgo biloba leaves, 2 cups of alcohol.

Instruction - You can make candies or a tincture – the choice is yours, and the benefits are the same! Check Chapter One for instructions!

 How to Use It – take it with meals three times daily, as a standard dose of 40mg (around 1 teaspoon).

30. ASTRALGUS ROOT (ASTRAGALUS)

 Medicinal Properties – It can reduce inflammation, increase collagen production, and increase skin elasticity.

 Fun Fact – Consuming astralgus root can help you sleep better.

 Why Will It Help – The topical treatment will reduce the redness and even the skin tone.

 How to Make It
Ingredients - a handful of dried astralgus root and some 80 proof vodka.
Instruction - Make a tincture according to the guidelines in the first chapter.

 How to Use It – Apply it topically to the skin using a cotton pad daily.

31. DEVIL'S HORSEWHIP (ACHYRANTHES ASPERA)

 Medicinal Properties – From skin diseases to stomach issues, this is a very powerful herb that can deal with it all.

 Fun Fact – It is also believed to cure toothaches!

 Why Will It Help – Because the anti-inflammatory compounds, as well as the antioxidant properties, can provide relief from dermatitis symptoms by preventing the infection, reducing the redness, and calming the skin.

 How to Make It
Ingredients - A tablespoon of the dried herb and a cup of boiling water is all you need.
Instructions - Add the herbs into the cup filled with boiling water and leave it for 10 minutes.

 How to Use It – After you leave it to sit for about 10 minutes, drink it.

DANDRUFF

A skin condition often overlooked by many, dandruff is one of the most common ones you will find. It happens to almost everyone at some point in their lives, and if you are currently dealing with it, here is how to help get rid of it.

32. HIBISCUS (HIBISCUS ROSA-SINENSIS)

 Medicinal Properties – It is known as the most beneficial herb for hair and scalp health. People mostly use it for hair loss, but it is used for dandruff, too. It contains Vitamin A, Vitamin C, amino acids, and other beneficial nutrients.

Fun Fact – Once picked, the flower of the hibiscus plant only lasts for a day or two.

Why Will It Help – Because it is rich in antioxidants, called anthocyanocides, and contains citric acid and malic acid, it fights off dermatitis by providing skin cell healing turnover and reduces inflammation and soreness. Additionally, hibiscus is a gentle moisturizer that reduces dryness and itchiness. All of these properties combined together can keep the scalp healthy and minimize the chances of dandruff.

How to Make It
Ingredients - 2 tablespoons Hibiscus petals and 1 cup Aloe Vera. Instructions - Combine them into a smooth paste.

How to Use It – Apply to your hair and scalp once a week, leave it for 45 minutes, and rinse with warm water.

33. HOLY BASIL OR TULSI (OCIMUM SANCTUM)

Medicinal Properties – It can calm the scalp, improve blood circulation, and reduce dandruff and irritation.

Fun Fact – Tulsi is used to cure fever and treat insect bites.

Why Will It Help – Because it will keep the scalp and the roots clean, avoiding excess buildup of dirt, which may cause an irritated scalp.

How to Make It
Ingredients - 2 cups of chopped holy basil leaves, 2 cups of water. Instruction - Bring the water to a boil and make a water extract as per the instructions in Chapter One.

How to Use It – Wash your scalp with it, then wash regularly with shampoo and conditioner.

34. BHRINGRAJ (ECLIPTA PROSTRATE)

 Medicinal Properties – Promoting hair growth is one of this herb's best Medicinal Properties . It also stimulates blood flow.

 Fun Fact – This herb can reach a height of almost 10 feet!

 Why Will It Help – Because improved blood circulation will lead to fewer scalp issues such as irritation and dandruff. Increased blood circulation promotes faster healing.

 How to Make It

Ingredients - a handful of the Bhringraj leaves, enough oil to cover them, 2-3 cups of water.

Instruction - Boil the water first, and then continue making an oil extract from it according to the instructions from the first chapter.

 How to Use It – Massage your scalp with the oil before sleeping.

Learning how to make herbal wonders to treat skin conditions is wonderful, but have you considered incorporating them into your daily lifestyle and improving your respiratory health? In the next chapter, let's delve deeper into the subject, uncovering some valuable information for you!

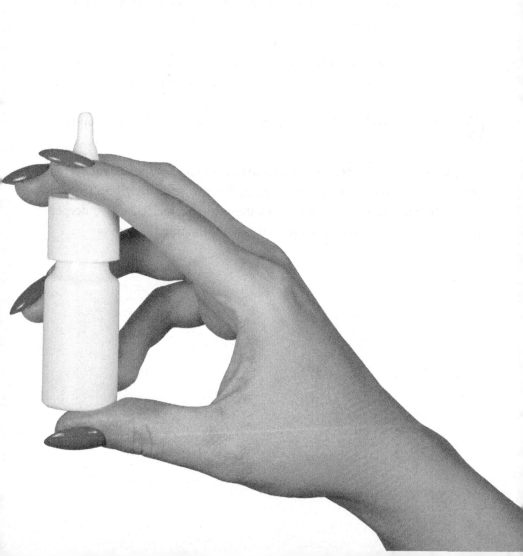

CHAPTER 4

REMEDIES FOR RESPIRATORY HEALTH

When pharmaceutical medicine reaches its limit, herbal medicine starts working its magic.

I have always found the longstanding history of herbal remedies and their many applications fascinating. Over the centuries, people have fearlessly tested the power of various herbs to uncover the vast scope of functions they have. That is why today, there is an elaborative list of incredible herbal remedies and their specific uses, including ones that can solve various respiratory problems.

Whether you are struggling with allergies, live in a very polluted area, or deal with respiratory viral infections and inflammations, in this chapter, you will learn how to implement the power of nature into dealing with common everyday issues.

Adding a little herbal magic to your home is exactly what you need. You can incorporate nature into your respiratory healing process in more than one way. Remember, the goal is to keep yourself healthy and do it with the help of as much herbal medicine as possible.

I was amazed by how simple herbs we know and use daily prove to have incredible capabilities. Discover all of them below!

HERBAL REMEDIES FOR COPD

Having lung issues is just as serious as having any other health issues. Most obstructive pulmonary diseases can be treated with a traditional medical approach, but there is no harm in trying out a few herbal remedies. And with any serious health concern, please do consult your doctor before making a wholescale change. Take a look below.

35. THYME TEA OR OIL (THYMUS VULGARIS)

 Medicinal Properties – It contains antioxidant properties that make it perfect for warding off any bacterial infections and relieving a cough.

 Fun Fact – In ancient Greece and Rome, thyme was seen as a symbol of power, courage, and strength.

 Why Will It Help – Because it contains antifungal and antibacterial properties.

 How to Make It
Ingredients – 1 teaspoon dried thyme, 1 cup of water.

Instructions – boil the water and remove from heat. Add the thyme and let it sit for 10 minutes. Strain.

 How to Use It – Enjoy a cup of thyme tea every day.

36. ENGLISH IVY EXTRACT (HEDERA HELIX)

 Medicinal Properties – Use this herb as an herbal remedy to help bring up mucus from the lungs, improve lung function, unblock any airway passages, and reduce swelling.

 Fun Fact – As a houseplant, it purifies the air!

 Why Will It Help – Because it provides anti-inflammatory and antioxidant properties and deals with cough-related issues.

 How to Make It
Ingredients – 1 tablespoon of the dried herb and 33 oz of water.

Instructions – Create a water extract. Check Chapter 1 under water extracts for instructions.

 How to Use It – Consume a cup daily.

37. GINSENG CANDIES (PANAX GINSENG)

 Medicinal Properties – Other than boosting your energy, it provides anti-inflammatory and antioxidant properties.

 Fun Fact – A dry pound of wild-harvested ginseng roots can sell for hundreds of USD.

 Why Will It Help – It will improve overall lung function because it has an antiviral effect against respiratory viruses.

 How to Make It
Ingredients – ½ cup of dried ginseng root, 3 parts water, and 2 parts sugar. Use these ingredient ratios to prepare a candy.
Instructions – Take a look at Chapter 1, under Syrups, Honey, and Candies.

How to Use It – Consume a candy a day until you feel better.

38. MULLEIN INFUSION (VERBASCUM THAPSUS)

 Medicinal Properties – This medicinal plant treats pulmonary issues, inflammatory diseases, asthma, COPD, and coughs.

 Fun Fact – Native Americans used it for rashes, bruises, and burns.

 Why Will It Help – Because the active ingredients in the herb can fight off the bacteria that cause respiratory infections.

 How to Make It
Ingredients – 1 teaspoon dried mullein, 1 cup of hot water.

Instructions - Make tea with this mixture. Take a look at Chapter 1, under infusions.

 How to Use It – Consume a cup daily.

39. HOREHOUND TINCTURE (MARRUBIUM VULGARE)

 Medicinal Properties – It provides some excellent anti-inflammatory properties, and it can prevent excess bloating in the body.

 Fun Fact – It is a part of the mint family.

 Why Will It Help – Because it will help you deal with your lung and breathing problems such as cough, asthma, COPD, and bronchitis.

How to Make It

Ingredients - ¾ cup vodka, ¾ cup distilled water, 1 ½ ounces horehound.

Instructions – Create the alcohol tincture as described in Chapter 1.

How to Use It – Consume 1 teaspoon daily.

40. WILD BLACK CHERRY TINCTURE FROM A DRY PLANT (PRUNUS SEROTINA)

Medicinal Properties – It can reduce inflammation and can deal with a cold, a persistent cough, bronchitis, and overall lung issues.

Fun Fact – When crushed, black cherry leaves smell like almonds.

Why Will It Help – Because it is a powerful cough suppressant and is especially useful for COPD.

How to Make It

Ingredients - ¾ cup vodka, ¾ cup distilled water, 1 ½ ounces wild black cherry.

Instructions - Create the alcohol tincture as described in Chapter 1.

How to Use It – Consume 1 teaspoon daily.

41. MALLOW LEAVES TEA OR COLD INFUSION (MALVA)

Medicinal Properties – In herbal medicine, it is a well-known demulcent (a soothing agent) that can deal with skin irritation and inflammation.

Fun Fact – It is filled with Vitamin C, Vitamin E, magnesium, copper, and iron.

 Why Will It Help – It can deal with COPD, dry cough, and a sore throat.

 How to Make It

Ingredients - 1 teaspoon dried mallow leaves and a cup of water.

Instructions - Put the leaves and the water in a small pot and bring the water to a boil. Then, remove from heat and let it sit for 5 minutes. Strain and enjoy.

 How to Use It – Drink one cup of the daily mallow leaves tea.

42. PLANTAIN LEAF TEA (PLANTAGO)

 Medicinal Properties – Enjoy its anti-inflammatory, antimicrobial, decongestant, healing, laxative, detoxifying, depurative, diuretic, antispasmodic, and expectorant properties.

 Fun Fact – They are known as "man's footprint" because they look like the sole of a foot.

 Why Will It Help – Because it is the perfect remedy for cough.

 How to Make It

Ingredients - 1 teaspoon dried plantain and a cup of water.

Instructions - Put the leaves and the water in a small pot and bring the water to a boil. Then, remove from heat and let it sit for 5 minutes. Strain and enjoy.

 How to Use It – Drink one cup of the plantain leaf tea during the day.

43. EUCALYPTUS TEA (EUCALYPTUS GLOBULUS LABILL)

 Medicinal Properties – It contains anti-inflammatory properties, which are excellent for dealing with COPD.

 Fun Fact – The eucalyptus tree can grow as tall as 250 feet!

 Why Will It Help – It will relieve the symptoms of COPD and fight off the persistent cough and congestion.

 How to Make It
Ingredients - 1 teaspoon dried eucalyptus and a cup of water.

Instructions - Put the leaves and the water in a small pot and bring the water to a boil. Then, remove it from heat and let it sit for 5 minutes. Strain and enjoy.

 How to Use It – Drink one cup of eucalyptus tea during the day.

HERBAL REMEDIES FOR ALLERGIES

Allergies can happen at any time – especially in springtime! Consider this your reminder to stock up on herbal remedies, and here are a few to get you started.

44. STINGING NETTLE TEA OR EXTRACT (URTICA DIOICA)

 Medicinal Properties – It contains analgesic, antimicrobial, astringent, and antioxidant properties.

 Fun Fact – Cooking the leaves removes the stinging effect, so you can even add it to a salad or a stew.

Why Will It Help – It has the power to reduce allergy-related inflammation without creating any side effects.

How to Make It

Ingredients – 1 teaspoon dried sting nettle leaves and a cup of water.

Instructions – Put the leaves and the water in a small pot and bring the water to a boil. Then, remove it from the heat and let it sit for 5 minutes. Strain and enjoy.

How to Use It – Drink one cup of the sting nettle tea during the day. Drinking it at night isn't recommended since it has a strong diuretic effect.

45. PERILLA SEED EXTRACT (PERILLA FRUTESCENS)

Medicinal Properties – Other than being useful in treating allergic asthma, it can treat sinusitis, nasal congestion, and eye irritation.

Fun Fact – The essential oils found in the perilla have an antidepressant effect on the mind and can boost serotonin levels in the body.

Why Will It Help – Because it can reduce the overall inflammation levels in the body.

How to Make It

Ingredients – 1 tablespoon of perilla seeds and some oil to cover it, along with some water (based on the oil extracts instructions from Chapter 1).

Instructions – Make an oil extract with the above ingredients. Find the instructions in Chapter 1, under oil extracts.

How to Use It – Consume only a few drops of it a day, diluted in water.

46. LUFFA

 Medicinal Properties – Due to its powerful antimicrobial properties, it is perfect for preventing colds and can do wonders in reducing nasal swelling.

 Fun Fact – It is grown in tropical areas and is part of the cucumber family.

 Why Will It Help – This versatile plant is often used to treat hay fever and can do wonders for your blocked nose, itchy eyes, and sneezing.

 How to Make It

Ingredients – 1 teaspoon of luffa, 1 cup of water.

Instructions – Brew a tea by boiling the water and leaving the luffa in it for a few minutes before straining.

 How to Use It – Consume 1 cup for a few days until the allergy symptoms disappear.

HERBAL REMEDIES FOR COLD AND FLU

The common cold and the flu are always present – what better way to get rid of them than the natural way? Here are a few herbs that can make all the difference.

47. SLIPPERY ELM LOZENGES (ULMUS RUBRA)

 Medicinal Properties – Its antioxidant properties help relieve any mouth, throat, and stomach issues.

 Fun Fact – Native Americans chewed on its inner bark to quench their thirst when water was unavailable.

Why Will It Help – It will help you deal with your upper respiratory ailment, such as a cough, the flu, bronchitis, and asthma.

 How to Make It
Ingredients - ½ cup of dried slippery elm, 3 parts water, and 2 parts sugar.

Instructions – This is best made as a syrup. Take a look at Chapter 1, under Syrups, Honey, and Candies.

 How to Use It – Consume a lozenge a day until you feel better.

48. ECHINACEA EXTRACT (ECHINACEA PURPUREA)

 Medicinal Properties – It has some powerful properties that make it a common remedy to combat viruses and the common flu.

 Fun Fact – The active ingredients in Echinacea are not water soluble, making it the perfect ingredient for an alcohol tincture.

 Why Will It Help – Ever since its discovery in the 18th century, it has become a more widely recognized herbal remedy many people use to fight the common flu.

 How to Make It
Ingredients – ¾ cup vodka, ¾ cup distilled water, 1 ½ ounces chopped echinacea root.

Instructions – Let's make an alcohol tincture for this remedy. Take a look at Chapter 1, under alcohol tinctures.

49. CINNAMON OR GINGER TEA & HONEY

 Medicinal Properties – Honey is an amazing antiviral and also has antimicrobial properties. This "old-wives tale" recipe really can help when you are under the weather.

 Fun Fact – One ounce of honey is enough to one bee's flight around the world!

 Why Will It Help – Not only will tea keep you hydrated, but the tea and the honey have antiviral and anti-inflammatory properties. The honey and warm water also soothe that sore throat!

 How to Make It
Ingredients – Cinnamon sticks, fresh sliced ginger, honey

Instructions – Boil hot water with fresh sliced ginger or a cinnamon stick (or both), let it steep, and then pour into a mug. Add honey to taste.

Now that we have explored keeping out lungs healthy, let's move on to that next very important system, the heart, and see what herbs can strengthen our cardiovascular system.

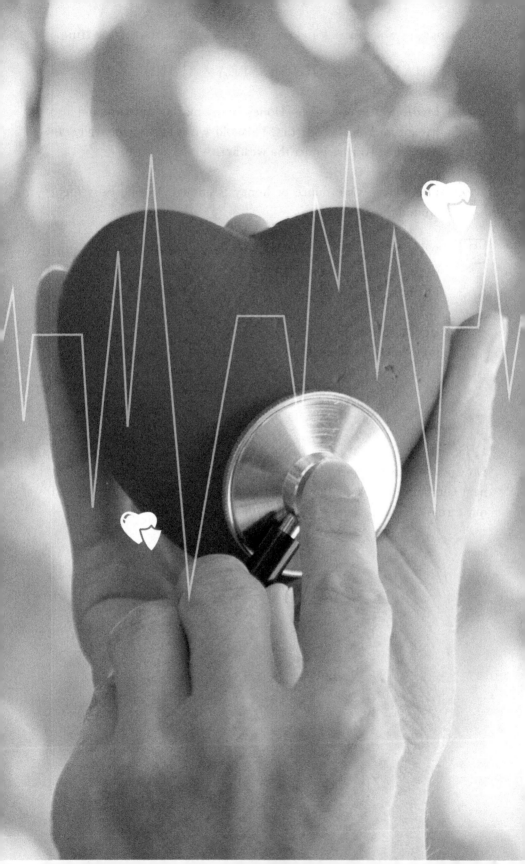

CHAPTER 5

REMEDIES FOR CARDIOVASCULAR HEALTH

The heart is the core of our bodies. It is the vessel through which blood is pumped to each part, and it is the wonderful organ that keeps us alive.

But, dealing with cardiovascular issues is a challenge in itself. It may disrupt everyday life, and living with a chronic cardiovascular issue can cause extreme anxiety over the loss of health and wellbeing. That is why many people tend to turn to herbal remedies.

Finding assistance in alternative medicine can be such a relief! Even if you are healthy as a horse, you may want to try these herbal recipes – they will fortify your cardiovascular health and help you maintain a smooth and balanced life. Being proactive with your health is the best place to start. And because we are talking about your heart here, a quick check with your doctor or naturopath is always advisable if you have a serious condition.

In this chapter, let's explore some of the amazing herbal remedies for cardiovascular health!

NOTE: Unless otherwise specified, the following remedies should be consumed daily

HERBAL REMEDIES FOR CLOGGED ARTERIES

There are more than a few herbal remedies that can assist clogged arteries. These have been considered some of the most popular and well-enjoyed products, so enjoy them and make them from the comfort of your home.

50. TURMERIC, MILK, AND HONEY SOLUTION (CURCUMA LONGA)

 Medicinal Properties – Turmeric contains curcumin, which is a bioactive compound. It can do wonders for your body, and other than presenting anti-inflammatory properties, it can prevent the formation of blood clots in the arteries.

 Fun Fact – Turmeric is widely used in cosmetics, too, because it is excellent for skin health.

 Why Will It Help – Because it will help reduce arterial inflammation and fatty deposits, making you as healthy as possible!

 How to Make It
Ingredients – 1 teaspoon of turmeric powder, 1 glass of milk, and 1 teaspoon of honey.

Instructions – Add the turmeric and the honey into the glass of milk and stir well.

 How to Use It – You can consume this solution once or twice a day to incorporate turmeric into your dietary plan.

51. GRATED GINGER TEA (ZINGIBER OFFICINALE)

 Medicinal Properties – Ginger contains gingerols, shogaols, and many other chemical compounds essential to the body's health, and they can effectively resist any cardiovascular complications.

 Fun Fact – Ground ginger root has a higher nutritional value than its raw counterpart.

 Why Will It Help – Because of its anti-inflammatory properties, it can reduce the effect of the free radicals in the body, improving blood flow and lowering your risk of clogged arteries.

 How to Make It
Ingredients – 1 teaspoon of grated ginger, 1 cup of water.

Instructions – Bring the water to a boil and remove from heat. Add the ginger to it and let it steep for 5 minutes. Strain and enjoy.

 How to Use It – Consume this tea once or twice every day.

52. GINGER, GARLIC, AND LEMON JUICE (ALLIUM SATIVUM)

 Medicinal Properties – Garlic is such a powerful remedy; it can destroy bacteria, parasites, and fungi, as well as lower blood pressure, sugar levels, and cholesterol levels, thus preventing blood clots.

 Fun Fact – The garlic can release its full potential if you crush it!

 Why Will It Help – Utilizing garlic can help reduce the amount of plaque in the arteries.

How to Make It

Ingredients – 1 cup of ginger juice, 1 cup of garlic puree, 1 cup of lemon juice, 1 cup of apple cider vinegar, 2 cups of organic honey.

Instructions – Extract the juice from the ingredients and put them in a saucepan. Cook for 30 minutes on medium heat while stirring. Remove from heat and let it cool off completely. Add the honey and mix well. Transfer to a clean bottle.

How to Use It – Consume 1 tablespoon of the mixture every morning, afternoon, and evening on an empty stomach. Keep the juice in the fridge for up to 2 months.

53. CAYENNE PEPPER DRINK (CAPSICUM ANNUUM)

Medicinal Properties – You may know that cayenne pepper has been used to treat stomach issues. But did you know that, because of its high antioxidant content, it can treat circulatory issues, too? It contains many vitamins, potassium, and manganese.

Fun Fact – Cayenne pepper is a type of chili pepper.

Why Will It Help – Because it can control blood flow, it can help the circulatory system and can strengthen the arteries.

How to Make It

Ingredients – 1 teaspoon cayenne pepper, half a cup of lukewarm water.

Instructions – Simply mix the cayenne pepper in the water, and your drink is ready!

How to Use It – Drink the mixture twice a day for up to a few weeks.

54. SOAKED FENUGREEK SEEDS (TRIGONELLA FOENUM-GRAECUM)

 Medicinal Properties – Fenugreek has mostly been used to slow down sugar absorption in the body. It is also used to reduce the risk of clogged arteries.

 Fun Fact – The fenugreek has a bitter taste. But, the bitter taste reduces when it is exposed to heat.

 Why will it help –Because it is believed to help the clogged arteries and lower the LDL (bad) cholesterol levels in the body.

 How to Make It
Ingredients – 1 teaspoon fenugreek seeds, 1 cup of water.
Instructions – Place the seeds in the water and let them soak overnight.

 How to Use It – The next morning, drink the water and consume the seeds on an empty stomach. Do this for at least 21 days to see significant results.

HERBAL REMEDIES FOR ARRHYTHMIA

An irregular heartbeat is usually connected to emotions. But what happens when there is something more in the background? You may experience shortness of breath, irregular pulse, heart palpitations, chest pain, and more. The important thing is not to take these symptoms lightly. If you want to do something to boost your heart health, here are a few remedies that can help.

55. ARJUN TEA (TERMINALIA ARJUNA)

 Medicinal Properties – This is an extremely effective herb against heart issues. It can protect the entire cardiovascular system, and it can fortify the muscles around the heart.

 Fun Fact – It is known to be one of the most effective herbal remedies for heart issues.

 Why Will It Help – Because it will strengthen and relax the heart muscles and provide the body with rejuvenating properties.

 How to Make It
Ingredients – 1 teaspoon Arjun tea, 1 cup of water, 1 cup of milk.

Instructions – Mix the water and the milk into a pan and then add the Arjun. Stir well and place the pan on high heat. Bring it to a boil and then reduce to low heat. Allow it to simmer until the liquid is reduced to a single cup. Remove from heat, strain, and add a sweetener if needed.

 How to Use It – Consume daily.

56. MOTHERWORT TINCTURE (LEONURUS CARDIACA)

 Medicinal Properties – Motherwort is an excellent herb that can promote women's health as well as heart health. It is the best herb to assist an irregular heartbeat, lower high blood pressure, and even help with anxiety!

 Fun Fact – The Latin name of this herb literally translates to lion's heart.

Why Will It Help – Because the main function of this herb is promoting heart health.

How to Make It

Ingredients – Enough motherwort to fill ¾ of a jar, enough alcohol to fill the jar too.

Instructions – Make a tincture of this mixture. See Chapter 1, under alcohol tinctures.

How to Use It – Use a few drops of it daily.

57. HAWTHORN BERRY SYRUP (CRATAEGUS MONOGYNA)

Medicinal Properties – Hawthorne has been used to protect the heart from diseases and control high cholesterol as well as high blood pressure levels. It can increase artery blood flow, improve circulation, and provide overall heart health.

Fun Fact – According to folklore, the Hawthorn tree is home to fairies.

Why Will It Help – Use the syrup to give a little bit of a boost to your heart, protect it from any health issues, and make yourself feel better in an instant.

How to Make It

Ingredients – 4 cups of fresh Hawthorn berries and 3 cups of brandy (this is for the tincture). Then, 4 cups of water and 2 cups of honey (this is for the syrup).

Instructions – Use Chapter 1 for instructions. Note – For every cup of syrup, use ¼ cup of tincture. Mix, strain, and enjoy.

How to Use It – Consume ½ teaspoon of it three times a day, either added to hot water or poured over ice.

58. HEART TEA RECIPE FOR ARRHYTHMIA

 Medicinal Properties – The combination of these herbs is such a powerful one that if you are dealing with heart issues or heart palpitations, or you just want to strengthen your heart, I believe this is one of the best one you will find.

 Fun Fact – This is the only unique heart tea recipe that will fortify your cardiovascular health.

 Why Will It Help – Because it will improve your blood flow and will help you deal with heart palpitations.

 How to Make It
Ingredients – 8 tablespoons of hawthorn berry, 2 teaspoons of rosemary leaf, 8 teaspoons of motherwort herb, and 12 cups of water.

Instructions – Combine together in one pot and boil to make a tea. Strain out the ingredients, saving the liquid. Fill your mug and enjoy.

 How to Use It – Consume daily for a healthy heart.

HERBAL REMEDIES FOR HYPERTENSION

Hypertension (or high blood pressure) is becoming a more common health issue with every passing day. Dealing with it can lead to having a prescribed treatment by your health provider. However, if you want to take things a step further, there are always natural remedies that you can use. Be mindful that you need to talk to your doctor before implementing them.

Take a look at some of the most popular herbal remedies below.

59. GARLIC WATER (ALLIUM SATIVUM)

 Medicinal Properties – Garlic can stimulate nitric oxide production, positively affecting blood flow and decreasing any pressure on the heart. It can protect the blood vessels and regulate blood pressure.

 Fun Fact – Garlic used to be given as a medicine during World War 2 to soldiers.

Why will it help? – If you want to maintain optimal cardiovascular health and manage high blood pressure, use the antioxidant properties the garlic can provide.

 How to Make It
Ingredients – 1 clove of raw garlic (crushed and peeled), 3.4 oz of water.
Instructions – See Chapter 1 for full instructions.

 Why Will It Help – You can consume it daily in the morning, before breakfast, on an empty stomach.

60. BLUEBERRY JUICE (VACCINIUM SECT. CYANOCOCCUS)

 Medicinal Properties – Blueberries contain a very high level of antioxidants and if they are consumed daily, they can work their magic on the entire cardiovascular system!

 Fun Fact – Consuming blueberries can make you smarter! They are excellent for brain health, too.

Why Will It Help – Because they will decrease blood pressure, they will assist in lowering the high blood pressure, and they will help you keep your optimal health.

 How to Make It

Ingredients – 1 cup of fresh blueberries, ½ cup of water, and lemon juice from ½ lemon.

Instructions – Put all the ingredients in a blender and blend until smooth.

 How to Use It – Consume this juice once or twice during the day.

61. HIBISCUS TEA (HIBISCUS ROSA-SINENSIS)

 Medicinal Properties – This is a very popular plant for people who want to lose weight – but this is an excellent blood pressure reducer, too. Hibiscus contains many flavonoids, which are excellent if you want to ward off high blood pressure.

 Fun Fact – The hibiscus tea is filled with Vitamin C.

 Why Will It Help – Because it is the best herb for lowering blood pressure levels. And remember, the darker the hibiscus flowers, the greater the effect!

 How to Make It

Ingredients – half a teaspoon hibiscus, 1 cup of boiling water.

Instructions – Add the hibiscus to the boiling water and leave it to soak for about 5-10 minutes. Strain and enjoy.

 How to Use It – You can make this tea once or twice a day and enjoy it. Make sure to allow at least eight hours between each cup of tea. Also, if desired, you can add some honey to the cup of tea.

62. MANGABA TEA (HANCORNIA SPECIOSA)

 Medicinal Properties – Mangaba is filled with phytochemicals. They provide many antifungal, antibacterial, anti-inflammatory, and antiviral properties.

 Fun Fact – Mangaba, roughly translated to English, means "good fruit for eating".

 Why Will It Help – Because the plant is filled with properties that can help with vasodilation, thus lowering the overall blood pressure levels in the body.

 How to Make It
Ingredients – 2 tablespoons of mangaba bark and 17 oz of boiling water.

Instructions – Add the bark to the boiling water and remove it from the heat. Leave it to sit for a few minutes, and then strain and transfer to a cup.

 How to Use It – Consume two or three cups of it a day.

63. HORSETAIL TEA (EQUISETUM)

 Medicinal Properties – Horsetail is a natural diuretic and it can eliminate the excess fluid from the body. Also, it is an excellent tea to lower blood pressure levels, especially for people who are dealing with fluid retention.

 Fun Fact – The horsetail tree dates back to 400 million years ago.

 Why Will It Help – Because it is extremely beneficial for the body. However, it should not be taken for more than 1 week at a time.

How to Make It

Ingredients – 2-3 tablespoons of dry horsetail leaves and 2 cups of boiling water.

Instructions - Add the leaves to the boiling water and remove it from the heat. Leave it to sit for a few minutes, and then strain and transfer to a cup.

How to Use It – Consume two or three cups of it a day.

HERBAL REMEDIES TO BALANCE CHOLESTEROL LEVELS

Balancing cholesterol levels is just as important as lowering high blood pressure levels. If you have been dealing with some high cholesterol and want to take a more alternative approach to it, then you can turn to some of these herbal remedies below.

64. GLOBE ARTICHOKE LEAF TINCTURE (CYNARA CARDUNCULUS)

Medicinal Properties – The artichokes are an excellent source of fiber and can help your digestive system. However, people are using them to address their cholesterol levels, due to their antioxidant, lipid-lowering, and bile-enhancing properties.

Fun Fact – The artichoke is one of the oldest foods known to humans.

Why Will It Help – Because the globe artichoke leaves can have positive effects on your overall cholesterol levels. They can increase the bile flow and aid in the distribution and absorption of oils and fats in the body.

80

How to Make It

Ingredients – Take a look at Chapter 1, under alcohol tinctures for the full ingredient list.

Instructions – This remedy is best as a tincture. Combine the ingredients, following the instructions in Chapter 1, under alcohol tinctures.

How to Use It – The recommended daily dosage is ½ teaspoon of the tincture three times a day.

65. MILK THISTLE SEED TINCTURE (SILYBUM MARIANUM)

Medicinal Properties – There are many Medicinal Properties that the milk thistle seeds can provide, but the best is that they act as a powerful antioxidant that can reduce inflammation, lower cholesterol levels, and restore proper liver function.

Fun Fact – Other than being capable of lowering the cholesterol levels in the body, it can protect the liver too.

Why Will It Help – Because it can reduce inflammation and lower the bad cholesterol levels in the body.

How to Make It

Ingredients – Take a look at Chapter 1, under alcohol tinctures, for the full ingredient list.

Instructions - Take a look at Chapter 1, under alcohol tinctures, for the full instructions.

How to Use It – The recommended daily dosage is ½ teaspoon of the tincture thrice daily.

66. SHIITAKE MUSHROOMS (LENTINULA EDODES)

 Medicinal Properties – Shitake mushrooms have many uses – you can use them to help lower the bad cholesterol levels in the body, boost your entire body, and even use them as an anti-aging agent.

 Fun Fact – The shitake mushrooms date back to 1209, making them the oldest known cultivated mushrooms.

 Why Will It Help – Because other than promoting healthy cholesterol levels, it can promote heart health and boost your overall immunity.

 How to Use It – Consume three or four shitake mushrooms during a week, and over a period of a few weeks, they can lower the cholesterol levels by 10-12%.

67. YARROW TEA (ACHILLEA MILLEFOLIUM)

 Medicinal Properties – Yarrow leaves contain anti-inflammatory properties and flavonoids. It have help fight a fever and has been known to lower the body's bad cholesterol levels.

 Fun Fact – Yarrow is a symbol of being courageous and says "I love you despite everything."

 Why Will It Help – Because it will not only benefit your cholesterol levels but will promote proper digestion.

 How to Make It
Ingredients – 1-2 teaspoons of yarrow leaves, 1 cup of boiling water.

Instructions – Add the leaves to the boiling water to make a tea, remove from heat, and let it steep for about 5-10 minutes. Strain into a cup.

How to Use It – Consume a cup a day, but as it is a strong herbal remedy, consult with a health professional before consuming the tea.

Having some homemade herbal remedies at your disposal that can assist your cardiovascular health can make you feel safer and healthier. Knowing that they are right there in your kitchen can give you the feeling of calmness and peace you want.

But what happens if you want to fortify your entire body, not only your heart? In the next chapter, discover the herbal remedies that promote immune health.

CHAPTER 6

REMEDIES FOR IMMUNE HEALTH

Naturally boosting your immune system is the best way to maintain your optimal health. For most people out there, strong immunity is one of the most important aspects of their lives – as it should be! We all live in an era where vitality and wellness are the center of our collective consciousness, and the world of herbal remedies shines right through as a possibility to boost overall health.

This chapter is a journey to your own immune system, and I hope I can help you uncover every aspect of it, provide ways to help strengthen it, and help yourself become a wonderful and healthy person! Consider the immune health remedies below as an innovative way to approach yourself. After all, alternative medicine is a treasure that helps you harmonize with what your body needs and your spirit wants.

With a dash of positivity and a hopeful outlook, let's dive right into the world of herbal remedies for immune health and start treating yourself with a holistic approach – from the comfort of your own kitchen!

These herbal ingredients are some of the best ways to nurture your body and put some emphasis on personalized care. Try a few (if not all of them) and create an individualized approach – this will allow you to explore each remedy deeper and feel the rich immunity benefits of every single one.

IMMUNITY-BOOSTING HERBAL REMEDIES

Using herbal medicine as a way to treat yourself can be easy – if you know what you're looking for. Some herbal remedies are exceptionally good and safe to use. To give you an idea of what you should be looking for, look at the extensive list below.

68. OLIVE LEAF TEA (OLEA EUROPAEA)

 Medicinal Properties – According to WbMD, olive leaves can help reduce cholesterol and glucose levels in the body, and it can deal with some microorganisms such as bacteria, fungi, and yeast *(Merically Reviewer by Poonam Sachrev on November 27, 2022 Written by WebMD Eritorial Contributors)*. Overall, it reduces the inflammation in the body.

 Fun Fact – In the early 19th century, crushed olive leaves were used to lower a fever.

 Why Will It Help – According to the National Library of Medicine, there are bioactive compounds in the olive leaves that include flavonoids, secoiridoids, and triterpenes, which provide a lot of health benefits and have antioxidant effects on the body. *(Seref N El 1, Sibel Karakaya, et.al., Nutr Rev. 2009 Nov)*

 How to Make It
Ingredients – 1 tablespoon of dried and crushed olive leaves, 2 cups of water.

Instructions – Boil the water and steep the leaves for about 10 minutes, making a tea. Strain and enjoy.

 How to Use It – Drink a cup or two of this tea daily to get the benefits from it.

69. GOJI AND ELDERBERRY SYRUP (LYCIUM BARBARUM & SAMBUCUS)

 Medicinal Properties – It has the ability to strengthen the cell walls and prevent viruses from inhabiting the body.

 Fun Fact – It is believed that goji berries can improve fertility.

 Why Will It Help – Because this syrup tastes amazing and acts as the perfect immune booster!

 How to Make It
Ingredients – ¼ cup dried elderberries, 1 tablespoon dried goji berries, 1 tablespoon rose hips, 2 tablespoons cut and sifted astragalus root, 1 teaspoon cut and sifted licorice root, 2 cups water, 1 cups honey.

Instructions – Create an infusion from the elderberries, goji berries, rose hips, licorice root, and astragalus root. Then, continue making the syrup as described in the first chapter.

 How to Use It – Consume 1 serving (1 tablespoon) a day.

70. ASTRALGUS MULTI-GRAIN BOWLS (ASTRAGALUS)

 Medicinal Properties – It contains antioxidants, and astragalus can protect the cells against damage.

 Fun Fact – You can add astragalus to soups, stock, and any other dishes you want!

 Why Will It Help – Because it will boost your overall immune system, help prevent a cold, lower blood pressure, protect the liver, and diminish upper respiratory infections.

How to Make It

Ingredients – 2 tablespoons cut and sifted astragalus root, 3 ½ cups broth of your choice, 1 cup mixed grains, 1 cup brown rice, 1 teaspoon seaweed seasoning blend, and some salt.

Instructions – Make a decoction with the astragalus root using the instructions from Chapter 1, and then mix all the ingredients except the seaweed in 1 liter of water (4.2 oz cups). Leave it in the refrigerator overnight. In the morning, add the seaweed and cook as usual, adding the salt last.

How to Use It – Remember this recipe serves 4 people. Serve in bowls and enjoy.

71. AMLA AND GINGER INSTANT TEA (PHYLLANTHUS EMBLICA & ZINGIBER OFFICINALE)

Medicinal Properties – Amla contains anti-inflammatory, antioxidant, anti-microbial, anti-diabetic, and hepatoprotective properties.

Fun Fact – If you sip water after consuming amla, the water will taste sweet.

Why Will It Help – Because it will help you boost your overall immune system.

How to Make It

Ingredients – 1 tablespoon powdered licorice root, 4 tablespoons powdered amla berries, 3 tablespoons powdered ginger root (to make the entire tea blend). 8 ounces of water with a teaspoon of the tea blend to make a cup.

Instructions – Add the ingredients to the water and bring to a boil. Let it steep for 10 minutes and then drink.

How to Use It – Consume 1 cup of this tea daily.

72. SIBERIAN GINSENG EXTRACT (ELEUTHEROCOCCUS SENTICOSUS)

 Medicinal Properties – The berries of the Siberian ginseng can protect the immune system during intense training, and it can give your body that extra little bit of support.

 Fun Fact – Even though it is known as Siberian ginseng (also Devil's bush), it is not really a ginseng, it is a woody shrub. People use it for many reasons – to treat a common cold or to enhance memory skills too!

 Why Will It Help – Because it will strengthen your immune system after it has taken a hit.

 How to Make It
Ingredients – ½ ounce amla berry powder, ½ ounce eleuthero root powder, 5 ounces vodka.

Instructions – Start by mixing the amla berries with the eleuthero root powder. Then, continue by making an alcohol tincture as described in the first chapter.

 How to Use It – A proper serving size is up to 30 drops of it three times a day.

73. IMMUNE BERRY ASTRAGALUS GUMMIES

 Medicinal Properties – These gummies are an amazing addition to all those who wish to add some vitamin intake but consume something that contains fewer preservatives.

Fun Fact – Gummies have become popular for adults, too – they are not just for children anymore.

 Why Will It Help – Because it will boost your entire well-being – and will do it in a fun way!

 How to Make It
Ingredients – 3 cups cherry/purple grape/pomegranate juice, ½ cup dried elderberries, ¼ cup cut and sifted astragalus root, 2 tablespoons amla berries, 2 tablespoons goji berries, ½ cup gelatin powder.

Instructions – Start by simmering the juice, elderberries, amla berries, astragalus root, and goji berries in a saucepan for 20 minutes. Then, divide the liquid into two cups. One of them can be stored in the freezer for your next batch, and the other goes in the pan along with the gelatin. Then mix everything until you get a thick mixture. Place in the fridge until solid and then cut into small cubes. Keep refrigerated until consumed. Use the extra liquid and when you need your next batch, add the gelatin and repeat the above process.

 How to Use It – Enjoy 3-6 gummies daily.

74. CINNAMON CORDYCEPS COCOA (CINNAMOMUM VERUM)

 Medicinal Properties – From antioxidant to anti-inflammatory properties, this is a beverage filled with health inspiring ingredients.

 Fun Fact – Cinnamon does not have a sweet taste, but it amplifies the taste of other ingredients.

 Why Will It Help – It has been reported to boost the functioning of the entire immune system.

How to Make It

Ingredients – 6 ounces of any milk, 2 tablespoons organic hot cocoa, ¼ teaspoon cinnamon powder.

Instructions – Warm up the milk and add the other ingredients.

 How to Use It – Pour into a mug and enjoy.

75. MAPLE GINGER IMMUNE ELIXIR

 Medicinal Properties – Bring balance to your immune system and helps deal with certain allergies.

 Fun Fact – Maples produces the best syrup.

 Why Will It Help – This gentle immune tonic is an excellent addition to your winter wellness repertoire.

 How to Make It

Ingredients – ¼ cup cinnamon codonopsis extract, ¼ cup holy basil extract, ¼ cup maple syrup, a small piece of peeled fresh ginger root, ½ vanilla bean.

Instructions – Put everything in a blender and mix. Leave it for a week before using it.

 How to Use It – Consume one teaspoon daily.

76. ASTRAGALUS CHAI TEA (ASTRAGALUS)

 Medicinal Properties – If one of your goals is to achieve a higher wellness state and improved system support, then this is the tea you should drink.

Fun Fact – Over 5,000 years ago in India, chai tea was used in Ayurveda, a holistic healing practice that focuses on healing through diet and energy balancing.

 Why Will It Help – It will help you healthily deal with stress.

 How to Make It

Ingredients – 2 tablespoons astragalus root, 10 slices organic licorice root, 2 tablespoons organic ginger root, 2 tablespoons organic dried orange peel, 1 tablespoon organic sweet cinnamon chips, 1 teaspoon white peppercorns, 1-2 organic whole allspice berries, 3-5 organic cloves, 6 cups of water.

Instructions – Add all the ingredients to a pan, bring to a boil, and then simmer for one hour.

 How to Use It – Add some milk and some honey to taste before consuming a cup.

77. ELDERBERRY SYRUP (SAMBUCUS)

 Medicinal Properties – The antioxidants and vitamin C found in this incredible plant can contribute to a healthy functioning immune system.

 Fun fact –Some people consume fried elderberry leaves.

 Why Will It Help – Other than being extremely tasty, elderberry syrup can promote resilience when the body is particularly stressed.

 How to Make It

Ingredients – 1 oz of dried elderberry, 4 oz of water, some honey.

Instructions – Bring the water to a boil, add the herb, and simmer for a short while. Continue using the instructions from the first chapter.

 How to Use It – Consume a teaspoon daily.

78. ECHINACEA TEA (ECHINACEA PURPUREA)

 Medicinal Properties – If you are looking for a healthy dose of Vitamin C, then this is the perfect tea to add to your list.

 Fun Fact – Native Americans have been using this herb as a remedy for centuries.

 Why Will It Help – Because it can boost the immune system, fight off a cold, reduce a sore throat, and clean sinuses.

 How to Make It
Ingredients – 1 tablespoon of dried echinacea root, 1-2 cups of water, a pinch of dried sage.

Instructions – Brew a perfect cup of tea by mixing all the ingredients.

 How to Use It – Consume a cup a day.

79. KOMBUCHA AND ELDERBERRY TONIC (MEDUSOMYCES GISEVII)

 Medicinal Properties – This mixture contains a high amount of antioxidants, Vitamins C, A, and B6.

 Fun Fact – It is a healthy alternative to a soft drink.

Why Will It Help – Because of its powerful antioxidants and phytonutrients, it will provide your immune system with a boost. Due to the antiviral properties of the elderberry and the beneficial bacteria found in the kombucha, your body will be able to fight any infection and inflammation.

 How to Make It
Ingredients – 2 cups freshly brewed kombucha, 4 teaspoons of dried elderberries.

Instructions – Mix the ingredients and leave it in a cool place for 2-4 days. Slowly open the bottle every day to avoid a glass explosion. Strain, store in the fridge, and use.

How to Use It – Consume a glass a day.

80. WATER KEFIR RECIPE

 Medicinal Properties – Kefir can help control cholesterol and blood sugar levels and help digestive health. It contains live bacteria that are beneficial to the body's overall health.

 Fun Fact – People consume kefir for glowing skin.

 Why Will It Help – Because you will feel lighter, less bloated, and healthier in your own skin.

 How to Make It
Ingredients – 3-4 cups of kefir, ¼ cup dried elderberries.

Instructions – Mix the ingredients and leave it in a cool place for 2-4 days. Slowly open the bottle every day to let out any built-up gases. Strain, store in the fridge, and use.

How to Use It – Consume a glass a day.

81. TUMERIC TEA (CURCUMA LONGA)

 Medicinal Properties – For thousands of years, turmeric tea has been used as a remedy due to its antioxidant, antibacterial, and antiviral properties.

 Fun Fact – Its active ingredient is curcumin, which is responsible for this tea's yellow color!

 Why Will It Help – Because the compound curcumin, found in this tea, will assist the digestive system and fight off bacteria.

 How to Make It

Ingredients – 1 teaspoon turmeric powder, a few ginger slices, a pinch of pepper, 2 cups of water.

Instructions – Prepare the tea as you usually would, and let the water boil along with the ingredients. Strain and consume.

 How to Use It – Consume a cup a day.

82. CINNAMON TEA

 Medicinal Properties – Cinnamon is filled with anti-inflammatory and antioxidant properties.

 Fun Fact – Antioxidants have the power to fight off the free radicals, thus minimizing the damage they do to the body.

Why Will It Help – Because it will help you control your blood sugar levels and your blood pressure too, will promote heart health, and reduce menstrual pain.

 How to Make It
Ingredients – 1 tablespoon of cinnamon powder, 1 cup of water.

Instructions – Leave the cinnamon to sit for 15 minutes in boiled water and then enjoy.

 How to Use It – Consume a cup a day.

83. LEMONGRASS TEA (CYMBOPOGON)

 Medicinal Properties – It has antioxidant properties that kill free radicals that wreak havoc in the body.

 Fun Fact – Lemongrass is known to quicken a person's metabolism.

 Why Will It Help – Because it will do wonders for an upset stomach, is helpful in treating an oral infection, and also provides antimicrobial properties.

 How to Make It
Ingredients – a handful of lemongrass leaves, a few mint leaves, 2-3 cups of water.

Instructions – Leave the lemongrass and mint leaves to simmer for 10 minutes in a boiling pot of water. Strain and enjoy.

 How to Use It – Consume a cup a day.

This was a chapter dedicated to all of you who wish to maintain optimal health at all times. It is important to remember that you need to take care of your body every day, not just when it is sick. Hopefully, you will find a few of these recipes useful – they will speed your metabolism and help keep your immune system in good shape.

Speeding up a metabolism is often connected to visiting the bathroom quite a few times during the day. But what happens when there is an issue with the body's drainage system? Read the next chapter to discover the herbal remedies for urinary tract issues.

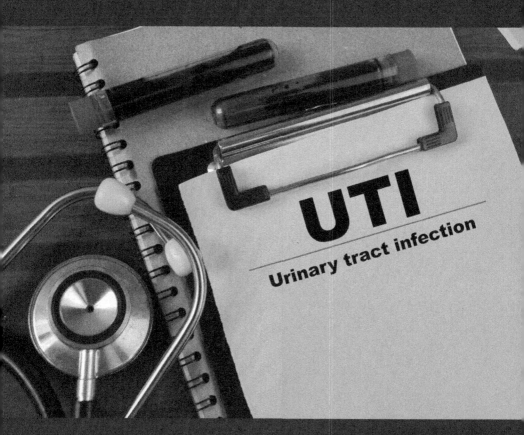

CHAPTER 7

REMEDIES FOR URINARY
TRACT SYSTEM

Taking care of your health requires a holistic approach, and by holistic, we mean considering every part and organ system of your body. Although often overlooked, the health of your urinary tract system is something you need to take great care of – and choosing natural remedies to enhance it is your best option!

In today's hectic world, one is bound to focus on finishing up their daily tasks on time. Having an extremely busy schedule, work obligations that cannot be postponed, and an active social life can lead to putting your health last.

With men, this results in low energy levels and even some minor health issues that they mostly ignore. What I want everyone to understand is to put yourself first. Turning to herbal remedies to give you that extra kick of health in your life can make a big impact.

The same thing goes for women, too. How often have you noticed something in your body is off – most likely due to hormones? It is of utmost essence to support your body through every change, and you can do that by adding some herbal remedies to your everyday life.

In this chapter, let's find out how to properly utilize herbal medicine to your advantage.

HERBAL REMEDIES TO TREAT UTI'S

For those of you looking to ward off UTIs, there are more than a handful of herbal remedies below that you can try!

84. CRANBERRY TEA (VACCINIUM OXYCOCCUS)

 Medicinal Properties – Cranberries are rich in antioxidants, especially anthocyanins and flavanols, which provide a plateau of benefits, improving several risk factors, such as cholesterol levels, blood pressure, heart disease, and, finally, UTIs.

 Fun Fact – Cranberries are native only to North America.

 Why Will It Help – Cranberries contain proanthocyanidins, which have anti-inflammatory properties and can help with urinary tract infections.

 How to Make It
Ingredients – 1 handful of dried fruit, 2 tablespoons cranberry leaves, and 4 ½ cups of water.

Instructions – Make a tea by boiling the water, then pour it over the leaves and fruit. Leave it for about 10 minutes, then strain.

 How to Use It – Consume a cup in the morning, noon, and evening!

85. UVA URSI BLADDER RELIEF TEA (ARCTOSTAPHYLOS UVA-URSI)

 Medicinal Properties – It provides antimicrobial, antiseptic, anti-inflammatory, astringent, and diuretic properties.

 Fun Fact – Another name for uva ursi is bearberry.

 Why Will It Help – Because of its antiseptic and anti-inflammatory properties, it can often successfully deal with urinary tract infections and cystitis.

 How to Make It

Ingredients – 1 oz uva ursi dried leaf, 1 oz dried nettle leaf, 5 oz dried rose petal, 5 oz dried marshmallow root.

Instructions – Mix all the ingredients and keep them in a cool, dry place. To prepare the tea, take one or two teaspoons and put them into a cup of boiled water. Steep for 5-7 minutes. Strain and enjoy.

 How to Use It – If your UTI persists, drink this tea up to three times a day.

86. PARSLEY TEA (PETROSELINUM CRISPUM)

 Medicinal Properties – The leaf, the seed, and the root are used to treat UTIs, help pass kidney stones, and treat gastrointestinal disorders, as well as constipation.

 Fun Fact – Parsley belongs to the same family as celery, carrot, and cumin.

 Why Will It Help – Because of its natural diuretic properties, it is the perfect home remedy to help you cleanse your body from infectious organisms and speed up the recovery of the bladder.

How to Make It

Ingredients – 1 ½ tablespoons of fresh chopped parsley leaves, 10 ½ cups of water.

Instructions – Boil the water, add the leaves, cover the pan, and let it simmer for about 5 minutes. Then, remove it from heat and allow it to cool down. Strain and enjoy.

How to Use It – Use it as a water substitute for one whole day only, and consume it at least every three hours.

87. PARSLEY TEA WITH CORNSILK (MAYDIS STIGMA)

Medicinal Properties – The Medicinal Properties in the cornsilk, such as being a strong diuretic and containing a flavonoid – an antioxidant, can help you treat inflammation in the prostate, UTIs, bladder infections, kidney stones, bed wetting, etc. Who know that there was medicinal benefits of corn silk... something we often throw out after husking an ear of corn!

Fun Fact – Cornsilk is a key part of the reproductive system of corn, making it an important factor for crop pollination.

Why Will It Help – Parsley, in combination with cornsilk, is one of the best herbal remedies I know for UTIs due to its diuretic properties, which flush your system and help cleanse your bladder from infectious organisms.

How to Make It

Ingredients – 1 tablespoon chopped fresh parsley, 1 tablespoon corn silk, 4 cups of water.

Instructions – Place the ingredients in the water and boil for a few minutes. Strain and enjoy.

How to Use It – Drink throughout the day.

88. DANDELION TEA (TARAXACUM)

 Medicinal Properties – Other than stimulating appetite and aiding poor digestion, dandelions have antioxidant and diuretic properties, too, which are helpful against UTIs.

 Fun Fact – Dandelions hold more nutrients than most of the vegetables you consume.

 Why Will It Help – Because of its diuretic properties, which will help increase urine quantity, thus flushing out bacteria and infection.

 How to Make It
Ingredients – 1 tablespoon of leaves and roots of a dandelion, 1 cup of water.

Instructions – Boil the water, then add the dandelion to it. Let it sit for 5-10 minutes. Strain.

 How to Use It – Consume it two to three times a day.

89. CELERY TEA (APIUM GRAVEOLENS)

 Medicinal Properties – Celery is a superfood rich in antioxidants, which has anti-inflammatory, antibacterial, and anti-viral properties. Some of the top health benefits of celery include improving memory, managing blood sugar levels, improving heart health, and suppressing inflammation in the body.

 Fun Fact – This vegetable is mentioned in Homer's The Iliad.

Why Will It Help – Because it acts as a diuretic, it may provide you with the UTI relief you are looking for. Paired with antioxidants, it helps fight bacteria.

 How to Make It

Ingredients – 1 cup of fresh chopped celery leaves, 3 cups of water.

Instructions – Boil the water, add the leaves, and simmer for about 20 minutes. Strain and enjoy.

 How to Use It – Drink 6-8 cups a day for the first two days, then reduce the amount daily. Consume a total of 8 days.

90. YARROW TEA (ACHILLEA MILLEFOLIUM)

 Medicinal Properties – Yarrow has antispasmodic properties, which makes it excellent when it comes to relaxing the muscles in the intestine and uterus. It will help reduce the UTI-induced pain and inflammation in the bladder.

 Fun Fact – Yarrow is a short-lived perennial that self-seeds.

 Why Will It Help – Because of its flavonoids and alkaloids, it can help with bladder infections, gastrointestinal tract discomfort, and even diarrhea.

 How to Make It

Ingredients – 1 tablespoon of dried yarrow flowers and leaves (fresh ones can work too if you don't have dry ones), 1 tablespoon of uva ursi, 1 tablespoon of cornsilk, and 1 ½ tablespoons of juniper berries. Additionally, 1 teaspoon of echinacea root for the concoction.

Instructions – Mix the above ingredients together in a small bowl. Prepare a concoction by simmering 1 teaspoon of echinacea root in 3 cups of water for 20 minutes. Remove from heat, add 1 ½ teaspoon of the above mixture, and steep until cool. Strain and consume.

 How to Use It – Consume a cup a day for 7 days.

91. FLAX SEED TEA (LINUM USITATISSIMUM)

 Medicinal Properties – Flax seeds provide an overall immune health boost. They have diuretic effects, so they are commonly used in cases of UTI.

 Fun Fact – Flax seeds are filled with protein!

 Why Will It Help – Flax seeds have lignan, whose chemical compound can alleviate lower urinary tract symptoms.

 How to Make It
Ingredients – 1 tablespoon of shepherd's purse, 1 tablespoon of flax seeds, 1 tablespoon of uva ursi, 1 tablespoon of echinacea root, 4 cups of water.

Instructions – Boil the water, add the ingredients, simmer for 20 minutes, then let it cool. Strain and drink.

 How to Use It – Drink 3-5 cups a day, preferably unsweetened, if you are dealing with infections that cause bleeding. Just a reminder that if the bleeding doesn't clear up quickly, see your health professional.

HERBAL REMEDIES FOR CLOUDY URINE

Cloudy urine can be the symptom of many issues – including kidney stones, infections, or other issues with your health. If you want to get rid of it, here are a few remedies that can help you.

92. GARLIC CORIANDER TEA (ALLIUM SATIVUM & CORIANDRUM SATIVUM)

 Medicinal Properties – If you want to deal with an infection caused by fungus and bacteria, then I have found that coriander is the best addition you can include from your kitchen. Because of its anti-bacterial properties, it can also deal with IBS, intestinal gas, constipation, and diarrhea.

 Fun Fact – Coriander gets its name from a bug.

 Why Will It Help – This is the best natural combination you can turn to to deal with cloudy urine. Both ingredients are anti-bacterial, and they keep bacterial infections away.

 How to Make It
Ingredients – ½ teaspoon of coriander, 1 big clove of garlic, 1 cup of water.

Instructions – Brew the ingredients in the water for a few minutes. Allow it to cool down, strain, and enjoy.

 How to Use It – Consume one cup a day.

93. GINGER JUICE (ZINGIBER OFFICINALE)

 Medicinal Properties – Ginger can deal with inflammation and reduce the risk of many infections in the body. It contains antimicrobial, antioxidant, and anti-inflammatory properties.

Fun Fact – Ginger has a therapeutic action that stimulates saliva production.

 Why Will It Help – Because it is an anti-inflammatory agent, it will keep your optimal level of health and diminish any infection that leads to cloudy urine.

 How to Make It
Ingredients – ½ inch raw ginger, 1 cup of water, 1 tablespoon of honey.

Instructions – Boil the water, add the ginger root (after chopping it up nicely), and leave it for 10 minutes. Strain and consume.

How to Use It – Add the honey (optional) and enjoy a cup a day.

94. BLUEBERRY JUICE (VACCINIUM CYANOCOCCUS)

 Medicinal Properties – Blueberries contain antioxidants, and they have the ability to eliminate the bacteria that cause UTIs.

 Fun Fact – One blueberry bush can produce up to 6000 blueberries within a year.

 Why Will It Help – Blueberries are rich in anthocyanins, which can help fight UTI. The juice is a natural urinary tonic that can deal with cloudy urine.

 How to Make It
Ingredients – 2 cups of blueberries, 2 cups of water.

Instructions – Put the ingredients in a blender and blend until smooth. Consume first thing in the morning.

How to Use It – Consume every day until the urine becomes clear.

95. PARSLEY JUICE BLEND (PETROSELINUM CRISPUM)

 Medicinal Properties – As mentioned before, parsley is a diuretic that can help eliminate any urinary tract infections and even kidney stones.

 Fun Fact – If you chew on fresh parsley leaves, you can eliminate your bad breath.

 Why Will It Help – Because it is a natural diuretic that increases urine output. This will help wash away harmful bacteria, clearing up irritation within the urinary tract system.

 How to Make It
Ingredients – A handful of parsley, 1-2 carrots or beets, or ½ cucumber.
Instructions – Add all the ingredients to a blender and blend until smooth.

 How to Use It – Consume this juice twice a day until your urine clears up.

96. CELERY JUICE (APIUM GRAVEOLENS)

 Medicinal Properties – Celery contains many antimicrobial properties that help eliminate the bacteria that cause UTIs. Also, it is an excellent source of iron and vitamins A and E.

 Fun Fact – Celery is a vegetable native to the Mediterranean region.

Why Will It Help – Due to its antimicrobial properties and being rich in antioxidants, it is widely used to treat urinary tract infections.

How to Make It

Ingredients – 4-5 celery stalks, ½ large cucumber, 1 inch-long piece of ginger, a cup of water.

Instructions – Add everything to a blender and blend until smooth.

How to Use It – Consume a cup daily until you feel better.

97. CORIANDER CONCOCTION (CORIANDRUM SATIVUM)

Medicinal Properties – Coriander seeds are known to be antimicrobial and anti-inflammatory, making them highly beneficial when treating a urinary tract infection.

Fun Fact – The coriander seeds have a warm flavor with a little bit of a citrus punch.

Why Will It Help – Because it will help lower your inflammation and fight bacteria in the bladder.

How to Make It

Ingredients – 1 teaspoon of coriander seeds, 1 ½ cups of water.

Instructions – Boil the coriander seeds in the water for 3-4 minutes, then strain and enjoy the decoction.

How to Use It – Consume this twice a day.

HERBAL REMEDIES FOR INCONTINENCE

When the muscles around the bladder start to fail, it is time for you to start doing everything in your power to prevent any urine from leaking through. That is when both traditional and alternative medicine collide to give you the best results. If you are looking for some herbal remedies for incontinence, then keep on reading to discover the best of them!

98. MULLEIN TEA (VERBASCUM)

 Medicinal Properties – It has anti-inflammatory effects, thus relieving pain and irritation in the body.

 Fun Fact – Native Americans used to apply this herb topically to treat skin issues.

 Why Will It Help – Because of its anti-inflammatory properties, it will provide a soothing effect on the urinary tract and will facilitate urination. It will also ease a nervous bladder.

 How to Make It

Ingredients – 1-2 teaspoons of dried mullein leaves and/or flowers, 1 cup of water.

Instructions – Boil the water and then pour it over the mullein. Steep for about 10-15 minutes. Strain through a cheesecloth or a coffee filter.

 How to Use It – Consume 3-4 cups daily, but consult with your health provider beforehand to check if it suits your condition.

99. DANDELION TINCTURE (TARAXACUM)

 Medicinal Properties – Dandelions are known diuretics, which can help eliminate bodily fluids.

 Fun Fact – The dandelion symbolizes resilience, hope, and healing.

 Why Will It Help – The antioxidant properties will help improve your entire immune system and strengthen the gallbladder.

 How to Make It – Ingredients – 1 jar, enough dandelions to fill 2/3 of it, enough vodka to fill in the rest of the jar.

Instructions – Add the ingredients to the jar, seal it tightly, and leave it in a cool and dry place for 6-8 weeks. After that, strain it and store it in small dropper bottles.

 How to Use It – Consume ½ teaspoon twice a day.

100. OREGON GRAPE ROOT TEA (MAHONIA AQUIFOLIUM)

 Medicinal Properties – Oregon grape has been used often in the past (and today) because of its digestive stimulant properties and antimicrobial properties, relieving the bladder and the intestinal tract from any issues.

 Fun Fact – The Oregon grape can be a great laxative.

 Why Will It Help – Because of the abovementioned properties, it will help you cleanse the bowel, help treat any infections, and strengthen the bowel too.

 How to Make It

Ingredients – 2 teaspoons of the dried root, or 1 teaspoon of the powder, 1 cup of water.

Instructions – Add the Oregon grape to the water, bring it to a boil, and then turn it down. Cover with a lid, let it simmer for 15 minutes. Strain and enjoy.

 How to Use It – Drink ½ cup twice or three times daily.

There is no better feeling than when you cleanse your body, inside and out! After knowing what you can do to make yourself feel better naturally, there's no stopping you! Once you try some of these herbal recipes, you will enjoy optimal urinary tract health naturally.

But your quest to enhance your overall well-being doesn't stop there – the following chapter is all about taking care of your muscles, ligaments, and bones.

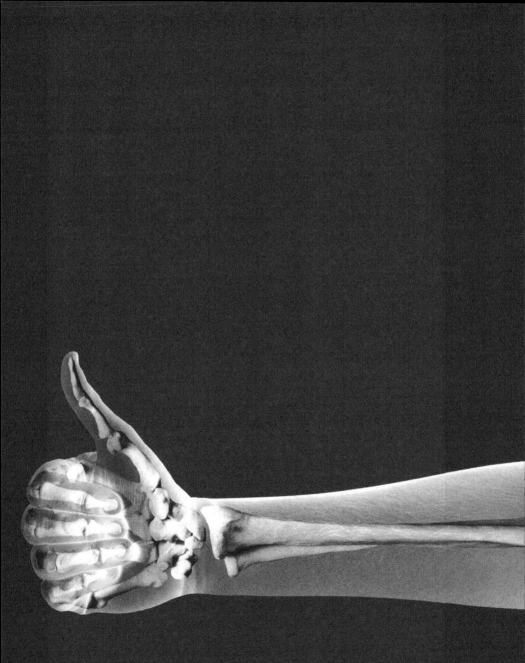

CHAPTER 8

BONE, LIGAMENT, AND MUSCLE HEALTH

Herbal medicine is for everyone – this chapter uncovers the wonderful secrets of herbs that can contribute to the health of the bones, muscles, and ligaments.

All of us are dealing with physical pain. Anything from smaller issues such as muscle pain to larger conditions such as arthritis pain – we have all had them at a certain point in our lives. If you have been one of the lucky few, you rarely experienced them. But, if you found yourself on the other side of the spectrum, then you must have already tried many different medications to soothe your pain.

I am here to tell you that there is a whole new world for you to uncover! In addition, let's explore some of the best pain management remedies for common aches.

HERBAL REMEDIES FOR ARTHRITIS

Let's start our exploration today with a condition that tops the "pain chart". Arthritis pain can be a mind-numbing feeling. Thankfully, there are many ways you can deal with it naturally. Take a look below!

101. ALOE VERA GEL (ALOE BARBADENSIS MILLER)

 Medicinal Properties – The highly moisturizing gel found in aloe vera leaves contains antioxidant and anti-inflammatory properties that can protect your skin from the damaging effects of the sun. Furthermore, aloe vera contains unique polysaccharides, a chain of natural sugars that have skin-healing properties. But it is the anti-inflammatory properties that make this a good addition to your arthritis management plan.

 Fun Fact – The aloe gel consists of 96% water, enabling the plant to survive in arid regions.

 Why Will It Help – Along with the medicinal properties come the vitamins A, C, and E, which reduce inflammation – thus helping your arthritis pain.

 How to Make It
Ingredients – 1 aloe vera leaf.

Instructions – Wash the leaf and stand it upright in a bowl or a cup for about 15 minutes, allowing the yellowish-tinted resin to drain out of the leaf. Then, peel the leaf. Scoop out the aloe vera gel with a small spoon and into a blender. Be careful not to add pieces of the aloe vera skin. Blend until it is frothy (about a few seconds). Transfer to a clean jar.

 How to Use It – You can use this gel for up to a week – apply directly to your skin daily in the area where you feel joint pain.

102.   CAT'S CLAW TINCTURE (UNCARIA TOMENTOSA)

 Medicinal Properties – It contains anti-inflammatory properties that can treat fever, fatigue, joint pain, and muscle pain, plus help reduce any chronic inflammatory symptoms.

 Fun Fact – This plant is a vine and can climb up to 50 feet high – or more!

 Why Will It Help – Because of its anti-inflammatory properties, it will minimize your symptoms of arthritis without significant side effects.

 How to Make It
Ingredients – a handful of the cat's claw and a clear alcohol like vodka.

Instructions – We will make this into a tincture. Add the herbs to a sterilized jar and fully submerge them in alcohol. Continue making the tincture as per the instructions in the first chapter.

 How to Use It – Take up to 25 drops of it orally, three times a day, with a little water or juice. Do not exceed the stated dose.

103.   GINGER POWDER OINTMENT (ZINGIBER OFFICINALE)

 Medicinal Properties – Ginger contains anti-inflammatory properties that help alleviate pain in the body. It successfully fights degenerative diseases, such as osteoarthritis.

 Fun Fact – Ground ginger root has a higher nutritional value than the raw ginger root.

Why Will It Help – Because of its anti-inflammatory properties, it will help ease the pain you feel in your joints.

 How to Make It

Ingredients – ½ cup of extra virgin coconut oil, ¼ cup of beeswax, 1 tablespoon of ginger powder, 1 tablespoon of cayenne pepper, 10 drops of lavender essential oil, and 10 drops of peppermint essential oil.

Instructions – Take a pan and add the coconut oil and beeswax to it. If you have a double-boiler, that's even better! Put that over medium/low heat. Once they are fully melted, add the ginger and the pepper. Remove from heat and let the mixture cool off completely. Finally, add the essential oils and mix well. Store in clean jars with a tight lid, and keep them in a cool, dark place.

 How to Use It – Use this topical ointment whenever you have joint or muscle pain. Do not take it orally, do not apply it to your face, and do not apply it to open wounds or cuts.

104. TURMERIC TEA (CURCUMA LONGA)

 Medicinal Properties – The main compound of Turmeric, curcumin, contains anti-inflammatory properties, thus helping you deal with stiffness and arthritis pain.

 Fun Fact – Turmeric is a cooking spice, so you can add it to your favorite savory recipes, too!

 Why Will It Help – Due to its anti-inflammatory properties, it may help alleviate your joint pain.

 How to Make It

Ingredients – 1 teaspoon of turmeric and 4 cups of water.

Instructions – Let's make a tea. Boil the water and add the turmeric – simmer for 10 minutes.

 How to Use It – Consume this tea daily.

105. WILLOW BARK TEA (SALIX)

 Medicinal Properties – It contains salicylic acid (also found in aspirin), making it an effective pain relief remedy.

 Fun Fact – Willow trees are a symbol of new life and fertility.

 Why Will It Help – Even if it acts slower than aspirin, it can provide long-lasting joint pain relief due to the salicylic acid.

 How to Make It

Ingredients – 1-2 teaspoons of ground willow bark and 8 ounces of water.

Instructions – Put the ingredients in a pot and boil for 5-10 minutes. Then, steep for 20-30 minutes. Strain and enjoy.

 How to Use It – Consume 3-4 cups daily to benefit from its use.

106. DIY ARTHRITIS OINTMENT

 Medicinal Properties – These powerful essential oils contain antibacterial, anti-inflammatory, and antioxidant properties, and when combined, they can help you experience less joint pain.

 Fun Fact – Coconut oil is the carrier oil that blends most easily!

Why Will It Help – Because the active compounds in the essential oils, it helps decrease the symptoms of osteoarthritis and rheumatoid arthritis.

 How to Make It
Ingredients – 20-30 drops of pure frankincense essential oil, 10 drops of pure ginger essential oil, 20-30 drops of myrrh essential oil, and 4 ounces of coconut oil.

Instructions – Put all the ingredients into a blender and blend until smooth. Store in a sealed clean jar.

 How to Use It – Massage the ointment onto all the areas where you feel pain twice a day.

HERBAL REMEDIES FOR MUSCLE PAIN

The human body is a magnificent and perfect machine. Each time something is wrong with it, it signals that to us via a certain form of pain. Muscles are no exception to it. Whether you move or sit a lot, muscle pain is the most common pain – everyone experiences it. Experiencing this a lot can make you turn to alternative medicine, and some herbal remedies can do wonders – discover them below and find out which ones work best for you.

107. DEVIL'S CLAW TINCTURE (HARPAGOPHYTUM)

 Medicinal Properties – This plant provides anti-inflammatory properties, and it can relieve pain and inflammation in the body.

 Fun Fact – This plant does not have an odor but tastes bitter.

 Why Will It Help – Because of its anti-inflammatory properties, it can help fight joint inflammation, muscle pain, and lower back pain.

How to Make It

Ingredients – a handful of the devil's claw, enough alcohol (vodka or gin) to submerge it.

Instructions – We are making a tincure with the ingredients. Add the herbs and the alcohol to a sterilized jar. Continue making the tincture as per the instructions in the first chapter.

How to Use It – Take about 20 drops of it orally, every day for up to 12 weeks. Consult with your healthcare provider for possible side effects.

108. ARNICA GEL (ARNICA)

Medicinal Properties – It has been used for centuries in homeopathic medicine because of its anti-inflammatory properties. It contains flavonoids, sesquiterpene, lactones, and phenolic acids.

Fun Fact – There are about 27 species of Arnica in the USA.

Why Will It Help – Because of its anti-inflammatory properties, it can help you with pain management.

How to Make It

Ingredients – 1 tablespoon of beeswax, 1 tablespoon of shea butter, ½ cup of arnica infused oil, 2/3 cup of water, up to 120 drops of one of the following essential oils – lavender, black pepper, jojoba, cedarwood.

Instructions – Boil the water and, at the same time, melt the beeswax along with the arnica oil and shea butter. Mix until combined. The water and the mixture should be at the same temperature – warm. Add the ingredients along with the essential oil to a jar, place your immersion blender at the bottom, and blend until smooth. Let it sit for 5-7 minutes, blend again, and do this until it stops separating when it cools down.

 How to Use It – Apply 2-3 times a day for up to 3 weeks. Never take it orally. This is a topical salve only.

109. CAYENNE PEPPER CREAM (CAPSICUM ANNUM)

 Medicinal Properties – It contains a compound called capsaicin that gives "heat" to your body. This means that the cayenne pepper can alleviate pain by heating the affected area. It also contains antioxidant properties, as well as many vitamins and minerals.

 Fun Fact – Cayenne pepper is a type of chili pepper.

 Why Will It Help – Because the heat can decrease muscle pain.

 How to Make It
Ingredients – 3 tablespoons of cayenne pepper, 1 cup of almond, olive, or jojoba oil, ½ cup of white beeswax.

Instructions – Melt the beeswax and mix the cayenne pepper with your oil of choice. Blend until smooth. Transfer to clean glass jars. Store in the fridge.

 How to Use It – Massage it daily onto the affected area to relieve pain.

110. CHAMOMILE ESSENTIAL OIL (MATRICARIA)

 Medicinal Properties – The chamomile is filled with antioxidant, anti-inflammatory, and digestive properties. Besides lowering your risk of several severe diseases, it can ease your muscle pain.

Fun Fact – Chamomile is one of the oldest herbs known to man.

 Why Will It Help – The 36 flavonoids that the chamomile contains all have anti-inflammatory properties – meaning you can massage this essential oil onto the affected muscles to relieve spasms.

 How to Make It

Ingredients – Enough dried chamomile to fill half a glass jar and enough jojoba oil to fill the rest of the jar.

Instructions – Place the ingredients into the jar and cap tightly. Store near a sunny window for 4 weeks. If necessary, open it to add some more chamomile. Sieve through a clean cloth into glass bottles. Use for 2-3 months.

 How to Use It – Massage your muscles with the essential oil every day.

111. CAMPHOR SOOTHING CREAM (CINNAMOMUM CAMPHORA)

 Medicinal Properties – It contains anti-inflammatory properties and is often used to treat inflammatory conditions in the body.

 Fun Fact – In India, camphor oil is popularly used in cooking.

 Why Will It Help – Because it will reduce your muscle pain and stimulate circulation at the same time by interacting with receptors on the sensory nerves.

 How to Make It

Ingredients – ½ cup of coconut oil, 2 teaspoons of beeswax, 5 drops of camphor oil, 5 drops of peppermint essential oil, and 5 drops of eucalyptus essential oil.

Instructions – Mix the other ingredients in a separate pot by melting the beeswax. Continue making the cream following the instructions from the first chapter.

How to Use It – Apply a small amount of the cream to the affected area and massage. Because it is very powerful, test a small patch of your skin first to see how it reacts.

112. HOMEMADE ARNICA SALVE (ARNICA)

Medicinal Properties – It is filled with anti-inflammatory properties, making it perfect for sore muscles, bumps, and bruises.

Fun Fact – Amish people are using it as a home remedy for chest congestion.

Why Will It Help – Because it will act as a natural pain relief for sore muscles due to its anti-inflammatory properties.

How to Make It

Ingredients – ½ cup of arnica oil, ½ cup of ginger oil, 1 oz of beeswax, 1 tablespoon of rosehip seed oil, 1 tablespoon of Vitamin E oil, 20 drops of lavender essential oil, and 20 drops of ginger essential oil.

Instructions – Add the arnica oil and the beeswax to a bowl and melt them on low heat. Once fully melted, remove from heat, allow it to cool down a bit, and add the other ingredients. Pour in clean containers.

How to Use It – Apply topically to the muscles whenever they feel sore or in pain.

113. CHAMOMILE HERBAL BATH TEA (MATRICARIA)

 Medicinal Properties – As stated above, chamomile is filled with antioxidant, anti-inflammatory, and digestive properties.

 Fun Fact – The chamomile bath will also help rejuvenate the skin.

 How to Use It – Because it has a soothing anti-inflammatory property that will calm your body down.

 How to Make It
Ingredients – A handful of chamomile flowers.

Instructions – Place the chamomile flowers into a cloth (in the middle of it). Then, take a string and wrap it around, making a tea bag out of it.

 How to Use It – Put it into your tub as you draw yourself a bath. Sit in it and relax.

HERBAL REMEDIES FOR BACK PAIN

I have been sitting in my chair for too long, and even when I am on a strict deadline or need to work fast, I still dedicate about 5 minutes every hour to light stretching. Not that I have chronic back pain, but I want to dismiss the possibility of that ever happening. If this is not the case with you, and you already experience back pain, then I present a few natural remedies for your attention.

114. CLOVE OIL (SYZYGIUM AROMATICUM)

 Medicinal Properties – This is the perfect topical analgesic – containing the same ingredient (benzocaine) as some of the most common back pain creams. It has anti-inflammatory properties, and it can help you manage your pain.

 Fun Fact – In India, the clove is added to some cigarettes and cigars.

 Why Will It Help – Because of benzocaine, it will help with the pain. Plus, you can use it whenever you feel back pain.

 How to Make It
Ingredients – 2 tablespoons of whole cloves, enough coconut or olive oil to cover them (not to fill the whole jar).

Instructions – Grind the cloves, place them in a small dark jar, and submerge them in the carrier oil of your choice. Seal the jar, shake it once a day, and leave it for a week. Then strain and keep the oil for up to 4 months in a cool, dark place.

 How to Use It – Use it in small doses and apply it to the back every time you feel inflamed.

115. CORYDALIS ROOT INFUSION (CORYDALIS)

 Medicinal Properties – This one has the perfect "pain killer" effect as it contains anti-inflammatory properties and alkaloids, too.

 Fun Fact – The corydalis belongs to the poppy family, and it has effective pain-relief properties right behind opium (except without the side effects).

Why Will It Help – Because it is an analgesic, sedative, and hypnotic, it can help you control your back pain.

 How to Make It

Ingredients – 2 teaspoons of corydalis root, ½ teaspoon of cinnamon, 2 cups of water.

Instructions – Boil the ingredients in the water for 5-7 minutes. Strain and enjoy.

 How to Use It – Consume ¾ cup when needed.

116. VALERIAN CORDIAL WITH WILLOW EXTRACT (VALERIAN OFFICINALIS & SALIX ALBA)

 Medicinal Properties – Valerian contains soothing, relaxant properties, allowing your entire body to relax.

 Fun Fact – Willow is where the salicylic acids used in the production of aspirin were originally found.

 Why Will It Help – Because of its flavonoids, it can help you deal with back pain.

 How to Make It

Ingredients – 6 teaspoons of willow tincture, 2 teaspoons of valerian tincture, ½ teaspoon of vanilla extract (to taste), ½ teaspoon of maple syrup.

Instructions – Mix the ingredients together in a bottle and store the mixture in a dark and cool place.

 How to Use It – Use up to 30 drops as desired, up to 6 times a day. This formula is for short-term use – until your pain stops.

117. TONIC OIL (CONSISTS OF CAMPHOR, PEPPERMINT, EUCALYPTUS, WINTERGREEN, AND FENNEL)

 Medicinal Properties – Any minor pain can be dealt with this way – this mixture contains antiviral, anti-inflammatory, antioxidant, and antibacterial effects and many nutrients.

 Fun Fact – Ancient Greeks believed peppermint can cure hiccups.

 Why Will It Help – Because of the combination of antiviral, anti-inflammatory, antioxidant, and antibacterial properties, the tonic oil is popular for relieving pain.

 How to Make It
Ingredients – 2 tablespoons of camphor oil, 2 tablespoons of peppermint oil, 2 tablespoons of eucalyptus oil, 2 tablespoons of wintergreen oil, and 2 tablespoons of fennel oil.

Instructions – Mix all the ingredients and transfer them to a clean bottle.

 How to Use It – Apply a little bit to the affected area and massage using a circular motion every time you feel pain.

HEALTH-BOOSTING HERBAL RECIPES

Now, giving your body an overall health boost is always a good idea! There are a few natural ways to do that, so here are a few recipes for your attention below!

118. GOTU KOLA DRINK (CENTELLA ASIATICA)

 Medicinal Properties – This is one of the safest herbal remedies you can try – it is filled with antioxidant, antianxiety, anti-inflammatory, antibacterial, and diuretic properties. Other than promoting exceptional memory, by promoting vitality and longevity, it can help you deal with your back pain issues.

 Fun Fact – Another name for gotu kola is Brahmi.

 Why Will It Help – Because of the antioxidant, antianxiety, and anti-inflammatory effects, it will relax your muscles and ease your pain.

 How to Make It
Ingredients – 1 ½ tablespoons of gotu kola, 3 tablespoons of dried milky oat tops, 1 ½ tablespoons of tulsi, 2 teaspoons of lemon verbena, and 32 ounces of water.

Instructions – Bring the water to a boil, then remove from heat, add the herbs, and leave it for half an hour. Strain and enjoy.

 How to Use It – Sweeten with honey or maple syrup and consume 1-3 cups a day.

119. FENUGREEK TEA (TRIGONELLA FOENUM-GRAECUM)

 Medicinal Properties – It has anti-inflammatory, antioxidant, anticarcinogenic, antidiabetic, hypocholesterolemic, and immunological properties.

 Fun Fact – Fenugreek tastes and smells similar to burnt sugar.

Why Will It Help – Its anti-inflammatory properties make it a particularly good choice when dealing with back pain, joint pain, and overall inflammation.

 How to Make It
Ingredients – 1 tablespoon of fenugreek seeds and 1 cup of water.

Instructions – Boil the water with the seeds, then let it simmer for about 6-7 minutes. Strain and enjoy.

 How to Use It – Consume a cup a day.

120. RHODIOLA HERBAL TINCTURE (RHODIOLA ROSEA)

 Medicinal Properties – Rhodiola is a known adaptogen, meaning it helps the body adapt to stress. It has antidepressant, antioxidant, and anticancer properties, too, and it is filled with nutrients.

 Fun Fact – Rhodiola was used in the past to increase endurance and work performance.

 Why Will It Help – Due to the antidepressant, antioxidant, and anticancer properties, this adaptogen will help decrease stress and improve your overall body function by diminishing pain. It may improve brain function and reduce signs of depression.

 How to Make It
Ingredients – A handful of Rhodiola roots and enough alcohol to fill the rest of the jar.

Instructions – Add the ingredients to a clean jar and seal. Continue making this tincture using the instructions from the first chapter.

How to Use It – Consult with your health provider for the correct dose, as every person and pain is different.

121. RED SAGE TINCTURE (SALVIA MILTIORRHIZA)

 Medicinal Properties – It contains anti-inflammatory, antiviral, and antioxidant properties. It can help you treat several concerns.

 Fun Fact – The red sage is in the same family as the mint.

 Why Will It Help – Because of the properties mentioned above, it can help you deal with digestive issues, stomach ache, gas, diarrhea, bloating, heartburn, loss of appetite, excessive perspiration, painful PMS, cold sores, asthma, memory loss, depression, high cholesterol levels, gum disease, sore mouth, sore throat, swollen nasal passages, and more.

 How to Make It
Ingredients – A handful of red sage and enough alcohol to fill the rest of the jar.

Instructions – Add the ingredients to a clean jar and seal. Continue making this tincture using the instructions from the first chapter.

 How to Use It – A commonly recommended dose is ¼ teaspoon three times a day, but you can consult your health provider to get the correct dosage.

THE IMPORTANCE OF EXERCISE FOR OPTIMAL BONE AND MUSCLE HEALTH

There is no strong body without proper exercise. Keeping your body active at all times means that you truly want to take care of yourself and be as healthy as you can get. If you want to maintain optimal bone and muscle health, then it is time to incorporate some exercises into your daily routine.

Exercise will help you maintain your health for as long as possible. It will have many positive results for your body, including the following:

- Improved overall quality of life
- Increased blood flow to the muscles
- A faster metabolism
- Reduced belly fat
- Lowered risk of bone fractures

When you exercise regularly, your bones and muscles will adapt, start building themselves up more, and become denser. Along with some herbal remedies, you will be less likely to experience a sprain or a fracture.

Together, we have combed through the world of herbs and plants and how to properly utilize them to ease a certain pain. Now, I am moving on to a more serious subject. In the following chapter, learn how to incorporate herbs to deal with and ease anxiety and similar conditions.

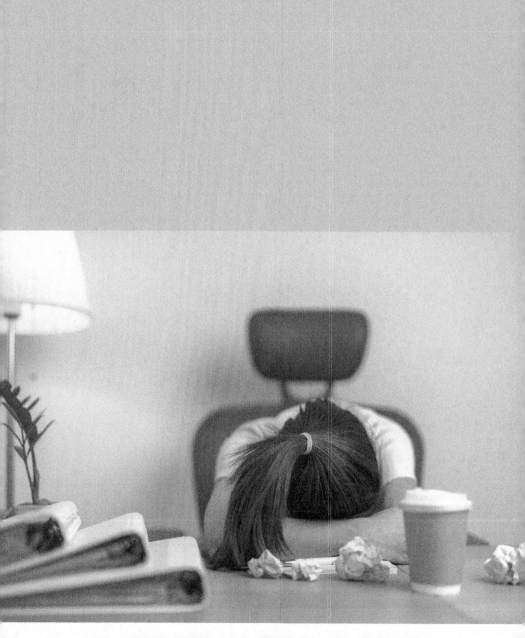

CHAPTER 9

ANXIETY

Occasional mood swings are a normal part of life, but that doesn't mean we enjoy them. Luckily, natural methods to enhance your mood are quite effective in lifting your spirits.

The power of a good mood can sometimes be a door-opener – both in professional and personal life. Keeping your spirits balanced is important. Also, let's not even begin to mention the number of people suffering from bipolar disorder, anxiety, stress, and depression.

So many people have turned to supplements that contain boosting properties. Medications such as antidepressants tend to come highly recommended. But are they always effective? And what happens when you don't want to take them but want to do something about your mood?

This is where herbal remedies come to assist. Many vitamins, minerals, natural herbs, and supplements can make all the difference. If you want to tackle this subject and naturally improve your mood, you are right where you should be.

HERBAL REMEDIES THAT REDUCE ANXIETY AND BOOST YOUR MOOD

As you are probably aware by now, anxiety is when you have been feeling stressed for a longer period. If left untreated, this state can lead to many serious health conditions. So, why not do what you can to diminish it? In addition, comb through the best herbal remedies that reduce anxiety levels and improve your mood!

122. MATCHA GREEN TEA (CAMELLIA SINENSIS)

 Medicinal Properties – Matcha is ground green tea leaves, and it contains enough caffeine to give you an energy boost. It also contains theanine, which provides a soothing effect – an excellent component to fight anxiety.

 Fun Fact – Matcha tea leaves are filled with antioxidants, too!

 Why Will It Help – Theanine will have a relaxing effect on the mind, will reduce anxiety, and will help with your concentration and focus.

 How to Make It
Ingredients – ¼ teaspoon of matcha, 2 ounces of water, 6 ounces of additional hot water, or steamed milk of your choice.

Instructions – First, sift the matcha in a mug to remove all the lumps. Heat the 2 ounces of water and pour it over the matcha – whisk until the matcha has fully dissolved. Add the 6 ounces of hot beverage per your choice and sweeten to taste (optional).

 How to Use It – Consume a cup a day!

123. ST. JOHN'S WORT TEA (HYPERICUM PERFORATUM)

 Medicinal Properties – This herb contains antiviral, antibacterial, and anti-inflammatory properties that can help boost the body's overall health. It also contains a compound called hypericin. Hypercin influences the action of the enzyme dopamine β-hydroxylase – which increases dopamine levels.

 Fun Fact – In the past, it was believed to provide protection from evil spirits and devils.

 Why Will It Help – The compound hypericin may help you treat anxiety, mild and moderate depression, and any sleep disorders.

 How to Make It
Ingredients – 1 teaspoon of dried St. John's Wort, 1 cup of water.

Instructions – Boil the water and then add the herb to it. Steep for 5 minutes. Strain and enjoy.

 How to Use It – Consume a cup of tea every day for up to 12 weeks.

124. VALERIAN TEA (VALERIANA OFFICINALIS)

 Medicinal Properties – The valerian root has been known for centuries to provide mild sedative properties.

 Fun Fact – There are records of valerian tea being prescribed for insomnia in Greece before the year 100.

 Why Will It Help – Because it will help reduce your anxiety, will tackle your insomnia, and will contribute to overall decreased stress levels.

 How to Make It
Ingredients – 1 teaspoon of valerian root, 1 cup of water.

Instructions – Boil the water and then add it to the herb. Steep for 10-15 minutes. Strain and enjoy.

 How to Use It – Consume a cup 30 minutes to 2 hours before bed.

125. LEMON BALM TEA (MELISSA OFFICINALIS)

 Medicinal Properties – It contains soothing and relaxing properties that contribute to the health and calmness of the body and mind. Bonus points for its amazing digestive properties!

 Fun Fact – Lemon balm can treat indigestion and menstrual cramps!

 Why Will It Help – The above mentioned properties can help you improve your sleep, reduce your anxiety levels, and act as the natural relaxant you need.

 How to Make It
Ingredients – 2 tablespoons of lemon balm crushed leaves (fresh or dried), 4 cups of water (the dose is for 4 cups of tea).

Instructions – Boil the water and add it to the teapot along with the leaves. Steep for 5-10 minutes. Strain and enjoy.

 How to Use It – Consume a cup a day for optimal results.

126. MACA POWDER (LEPIDIUM MEYENII)

 Medicinal Properties – This one is considered a powerful adaptogenic plant, meaning it gives the body powder to adapt and resist what's going on in it – such as depression, anxiety, and stress.

 Fun Fact – Maca powder is native to Peru.

Why Will It Help – Because of its adaptogenic properties, it can help you deal with stress and anxiety.

How to Make It

Ingredients – 4 tablespoons of maca root powder, 2 tablespoons of ashwagandha root powder, 2 tablespoons of astragalus root powder, 2 tablespoons of eleuthero root powder, and 1 tablespoon of licorice root powder.

Instructions – Combine all of them into a glass jar and add a teaspoon of the mixture to any recipe you want.

How to Use It – Use a teaspoon in your food recipes daily to boost your body.

127. BRAHMI POWDER AND MILK (BACOPA MONNIERI)

Medicinal Properties – This is the ultimate happiness ingredient! It is known for providing memory-enhancing abilities, it is an adaptogenic herb, and it has a cooling energy.

Fun Fact – It is named after Lord Brahma, the Hindu god of creation.

Why will it help? – The adaptogenic properties will help you deal with stress, and it will also help you improve your concentration and attention.

How to Make It

Ingredients – ½ teaspoon of Brahmi, ½ teaspoon of ashwagandha, 1 cup of milk.
Instructions – Warm the milk, add the ingredients and enjoy.

How to Use It – De-stress by consuming a cup of this beverage daily.

128. JATAMANSI ROOT INFUSION (NARDOSTACHYS JATAMANSI)

 Medicinal Properties – Jatamansi is a potent immunity booster. It contains sleep-inducing, anti-inflammatory, laxative, antioxidant, and antifungal properties.

 Fun fact: Other than being considered the perfect brain tonic, it helps prevent wrinkles.

 Why Will It Help – Because of the above properties, it will boost your body, reducing stress and fatigue. Consumption of this herb is connected to improved brain function and memory retention.

 How to Make It
Ingredients – 2 teaspoons of Jatamansi root powder, 1 large cup of water.

Instructions – Boil the water, transfer to a cup, add the powder, and allow it to infuse. Check the first chapter to see how to make an infusion.

 How to Use It – Consume a cup of this infusion any time of the day.

129. SHATAVARI TEA (ASPARAGUS RACEMOSUS)

 Medicinal Properties – it contains anti-inflammatory and antioxidant properties, boosting your overall immune system and calming the mind and spirit.

 Fun Fact – This is a species of asparagus native to Africa and Southern Asia.

Why will it help? – The anti-inflammatory and antioxidant properties can help you balance your emotions, reduce your anxiety levels, and promote an overall sense of well-being.

How to Make It

Ingredients – 1 teaspoon of powdered Shatavari root and 8 ounces of water.

Instructions – Brew the tea as usual by boiling the water and then allowing the herb to steep in it for a few minutes.

How to Use It – Make this tea and consume a cup twice a day.

130. TULSI AGUA FRESCA (OCIMUM SANCTUM)

Medicinal Properties – It contains antimicrobial, antioxidant, anti-inflammatory, anti-diarrheal, and many other properties, making it such a unique combination that people have been using it for everything!

Fun Fact – Tulsi is considered a sacred herb in India.

Why Will It Help – Because of the unique properties mentioned above, it can uplift your mood and balance the influence on the nervous system.

How to Make It

Ingredients – 2-4 teaspoons of fresh tulsi leaves, finely chopped, ½ cup of seasonal fruit of your choice, and 1 quart of water.

Instructions – Add the water to a pitcher, prep the fruit by cutting it into small pieces, and add the tulsi leaves to it, too. Leave it overnight or for at least 4 hours.

How to Use It – Pour into a glass and enjoy every day. Discard the leftovers after two days.

131. SMALL MEASURE OF CALM HONEY

 Medicinal Properties – Many antioxidant, anti-anxiety, and apoptogenic properties come with this mix.

 Fun Fact – Honey can be stored for eternity.

 Why Will It Help – Due to its antioxidant, anti-anxiety, and apoptogenic properties, it will act as a mood booster, supporting your nervous system and keeping anxiety at bay.

 How to Make It
Ingredients – 2 tablespoons of powdered goji berries, 2 tablespoons of powdered Schisandra berries, 2 tablespoons of powdered holy basil, and 1 cup of honey.

Instructions – Stir the powdered ingredients until you create an even blend. Add the honey and mix well. Transfer to a tightly sealed jar and keep in the fridge. This mixture lasts up to 6 months, but try to consume it within the first three months for freshness.

How to Use It – Consume a teaspoon a day.

132. HAPPY DAYS ELIXIR

 Medicinal Properties – Another mixture that contains adaptogenic properties and will work perfectly for the overall health of your body!

 Fun Fact – This elixir can help you if you feel a bit out of sorts!

Why Will It Help – Because it will act as an uplifting mood tonic and support your immune system.

How to Make It

Ingredients – 1/3 ounce of Rhodiola root powder, 1/3 ounce of eleuthero powder, 1/3 ounce of Schisandra powder, 5 ounces of brandy, and 5 ounces of honey.

Instructions – Add all the powdered ingredients and the brandy into a glass jar. Seal tight and gently shake. Leave it for two weeks (shake it every day). After two weeks, strain out the powdered herbs, add the honey, and bottle your elixir.

How to Use It – Consume 40-80 drops thrice daily. If it interferes with your sleep, only consume it in the morning.

133. ANXIETY TINCTURE

Medicinal Properties – This is an incredibly relaxing blend that will calm your nerves down.

Fun Fact – In California, the 6th of April is designated as California Poppy Day!

Why will it help? – Because of the valerian root, poppy seeds, and passionflower, it has sedative properties that will help you deal with debility and reduce stress levels.

How to Make It

Ingredients – 2 parts Valerian root, 1 part California poppy (leaf, seed, and flower), 1 part passionflower, and enough alcohol to cover them.

Instructions – Add the herbs and the alcohol to a jar, and continue creating the tincture as described in the first chapter.

How to Use It – Consume ½ to 1 teaspoon thrice daily.

134. PASSIONFLOWER TEA (PASSIFLORACEAE)

 Medicinal Properties – There is a chemical in the passionflower called gamma-aminobutyric acid (abbreviated GABA), which has been thought to have some therapeutic properties on the mind.

 Fun Fact – The name of this plant derives from travelers from the 16th century who believed that different parts of the flower symbolized the passion of Christ.

 Why Will It Help – GABA is a neurotransmitter that relaxes the central nervous system – it will help you increase your resilience to stress, thus promoting restful sleep, calm focus, positive mood, and an overall sense of well-being.

 How to Make It
Ingredients – 1-2 teaspoons of dried passion flower and 8 ounces of water.

Instructions – Boil the water and pour it over the herb, allowing it to steep for 30 minutes. Strain and drink 4 oz. up to four times a day.

 How to Use It – Consume a cup of this tea before bed to support sleep or during the day to lift your mood and decrease your stress.

135. KAVA KAVA DRINK (PIPER METHYSTICUM)

 Medicinal Properties – It contains relaxing and soothing properties, which can help you deal with your insomnia and disrupted sleeping schedule.

Fun Fact – The Latin name, loosely translated, means intoxicating pepper.

 Why Will It Help – Being a powerful medicine with relaxing properties, it can treat your anxiety and help you sleep better to feel refreshed the next day.

 How to Make It

Ingredients – 2 teaspoons of kava root, 2 cups of water, juice of one lemon, ½ a piece of ginger root, and a pinch of sea salt.

Instructions – Blend the kava and the ginger with the water. Add the lemon juice – then strain. Add the sea salt. This makes up for two servings.

 How to Use It – Consume a cup in the evening, before going to bed, and leave the other cup for the next night.

136. BATH BOMB

 Medicinal Properties – There is more to this bath bomb than the calming benefits – other than calming your body, it will calm down your mind, too.

 Fun Fact – Epsom salt can help you feel physically better.

 Why Will It Help – Because it will contribute to an extra-relaxing experience due to its calming effect and will contribute to an improved mental and emotional state.

 How to Make It

Ingredients – 1 cup of baking soda, ½ cup of cornstarch, ½ cup of citric acid, ½ cup of Epsom salt, 3 teaspoons of water, 3 teaspoons of coconut oil (melted), a few drops of essential oil of your choosing, dried lavender, and food coloring.

Instructions – Mix all the ingredients and add them to two bath bomb molds. Allow them to dry overnight.

 How to Use It – Add it to your tub next time you are drawing yourself a hot bath!

137. CHAMOMILE AND GINGER HERBAL TEA (MATRICARIA & ZINGIBER OFFICINALE)

 Medicinal Properties – Both the chamomile and the ginger will provide some calming effects on the body and relaxing benefits. The ginger contains gingerol, a main bioactive compound, which gives this root its anti-inflammatory and antioxidant properties.

 Fun Fact – The old word for ginger is gingifer.

 Why Will It Help – Because this blend packed with antioxidants and soothing properties will calm down the nervous system, relax the body, improve your sleep, and help with muscle spasms, too.

 How to Make It
Ingredients – 1-inch ginger root, 2 tablespoons of dried chamomile flowers, 3 cups of water.

Instructions – Boil the water, add the ingredients, and steep for 15 minutes. Strain and enjoy.

 How to Use It – Consume a cup a day.

138. AFTERNOON ANXIETY RELIEF

 Medicinal Properties – This tea will provide instant relief, as the Medicinal Properties include an incredibly calming effect – especially because it contains peppermint and chamomile – both with soothing properties.

 Fun Fact – Essential oils of chamomile are exclusively used in cosmetics.

 Why Will It Help – Because of its calming effects, this is the perfect anti-anxiety afternoon tea to sip on.

 How to Make It
Ingredients – 4 cups of water, 3 tablespoons of peppermint, 3 tablespoons of chamomile, 1 teaspoon of grated fresh ginger, and 2 slices of lemon.

Instructions – Boil the water and add all the ingredients inside. Steep for 15 minutes. Strain and enjoy.

 How to Use It – Consume a cup daily.

139. REALM OF RELAXATION

 Medicinal Properties – The ingredients in this tea mixture (especially lavender and lemon balm) provide mild sedative properties.

 Fun Fact – The orange trees were first grown in China.

 Why Will It Help – Because of the sedative properties, you will be able to deal with your insomnia, stress, anxiety, and even your headache.

How to Make It

Ingredients – 4 cups of boiling water, 3 tablespoons of lavender, 3 tablespoons of lemon balm, 3 teaspoons of honey, and 1 teaspoon of orange tree flower water.

Instructions – Boil the water and add all the ingredients inside. Steep for 15 minutes. Strain and enjoy.

How to Use It – Consume a cup a day before sleeping.

AROMATHERAPY ANTI-ANXIETY REMEDIES

For all of you who want to take it a step further and start enjoying the benefits of aromatherapy, a few remedies can help you achieve that. Consider preparing the ones below and enjoy a healthier you.

140. BERGAMOT, SAGE, AND LAVENDER BLEND (CITRUS BERGAMIA, SALVIA OFFICINALIS & LAVANDULA)

Medicinal Properties – When combined, these ingredients produce a decent amount of the Linalyl Acetate compound, a stress-relief agent.

Fun Fact – The sage is native to the northern Mediterranean.

Why Will It Help – Because it will help you in stressful situations and when you feel the onset of depression and anxiety.

How to Make It

Ingredients – 2 drops of bergamot essential oil, 2 drops of clary sage essential oil, 1 drop of lavender essential oil.

Instructions – Mix all the ingredients together and transfer them to a small glass bottle.

How to Use It – Add a few drops to your infuser or air freshener.

141. SANDALWOOD AND BERGAMOT BLEND (SANTALUM ALBUM & CITRUS BERGAMIA)

Medicinal Properties – Sandalwood contains antioxidant, anti-microbial, anti-inflammatory, and anti-proliferative properties.

Fun Fact – There are about 25 different species of sandalwood in the world.

Why Will It Help – Because of the abovementioned properties, it will help you soothe your anxiety.

How to Make It

Ingredients – 2 drops of sandalwood essential oil and 2 drops of bergamot essential oil (you can increase the dose; just keep the parts equal).

Instructions – Mix all the ingredients together and transfer them to a small glass bottle.

How to Use It – Add a few drops to your infuser or your air freshener.

142. ROMAN CHAMOMILE, PETITGRAIN, AND ATLAS CEDARWOOD BLEND (CHAMAEMELUM NOBILE, CITRUS AURANTIUM & CEDRUS ATLANTICA)

 Medicinal Properties – Use this essential oil blend to feel instantly calming.

 Fun Fact – Because of the strong scent, Atlas cedarwood is used in lining the insides of chests and wardrobes.

 Why Will It Help – Because it will help you combat the feelings of anxiety and will bring an overall sense of balance.

 How to Make It

Ingredients – 2 drops of Roman chamomile essential oil, 2 drops of petitgrain essential oil, and 1 drop of Atlas cedarwood essential oil.

Instructions – Mix all the ingredients together and transfer them to a small glass bottle.

 How to Use It – Add a few drops to your infuser or your air freshener.

143. MANDARIN AND ROSE ESSENTIAL OIL BLEND (CITRUS RETICULATA & ROSA RUBIGINOSA)

 Medicinal Properties – This is a powerful essential oil blend that comes with calming effects.

 Fun Fact – All varieties of roses are edible.

 Why Will It Help – Because it has a calming effect, this blend can help you ground yourself and reduce your anxiety.

How to Make It

Ingredients – 2 drops of mandarin essential oil, 1 drop of rose essential oil, 1 drop of lavender essential oil, and 1 drop of vetiver essential oil.

Instructions – Mix all the ingredients and transfer them to a small glass bottle.

How to Use It – Add a few drops to your infuser or air freshener.

If you want to calm down your nerves, this is the best way to do it. Remember to always practice kindness toward yourself. No matter your age, you should dedicate some time to yourself and do whatever it takes. Taking care of yourself is important – what happens when you notice there is a specific issue that only professionals can understand?

I am talking about diabetes – and the following chapter is all about specific herbal remedies that concern that particular health condition.

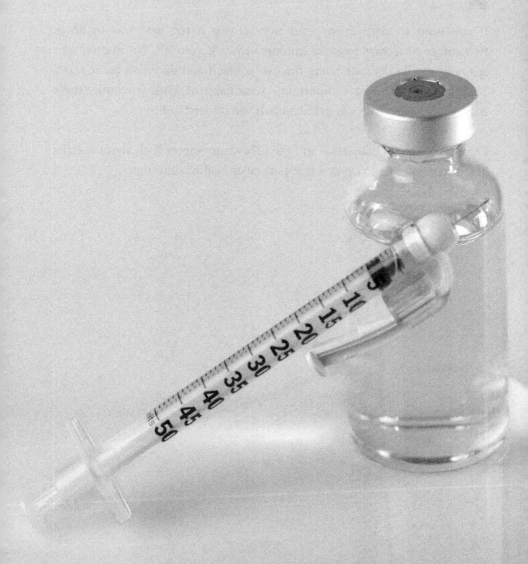

CHAPTER 10

DIABETES

Diabetes is a serious health condition that can happen to anyone. It is an issue that many people all over the world face – and some do it better than others. Have you ever thought about why that is?

The truth is, those who deal better with this condition did not achieve it overnight. Over time, besides the medication you take, you will learn that there are more aspects to it than one. The first thing you should focus on is adding a few herbal remedies. As many spices and herbs are known to have extremely powerful properties, some of them can assist in improving the blood glucose levels in the body. These are useful for people with a higher risk or already dealing with diabetes.

Include some of the best natural remedies to help you manage this condition and lead a healthier and more fulfilled life. I have picked the best of the best, just for you!

Herbal remedies to lower blood sugar levels

Diabetes can happen to anyone – a young or an old person, and it is a condition that requires constant care and attention. Sometimes, when you want to take that extra step in the process of caring for yourself, you might turn to a natural remedy. Here are a few to begin with.

144. BRAZILIAN ORCHID TREE LEAF EXTRACT (BAUHINIA FORFICATA)

 Medicinal Properties – It contains antioxidant, anti-inflammatory, anticancer, anti-microbial, diuretic, anticholesterolemic, and hypoglycaemic properties. It also acts as a blood purifier. The leaves contain alkaloids, flavonoids, and glycosides.

 Fun Fact – This plant is also called "vegetable insulin".

 Why Will It Help – When all these medicinal properties are combined, you get a perfect treatment for diabetes. Since this was discovered at the beginning of the 20th century, people have been consuming it for its ability to reduce blood sugar levels.

 How to Make It
Ingredients – 2 leaves of the Brazilian orchid tree, 400 ml of water.

Instructions – Wash the leaves, chop them, and then add them to a pot of water that has boiled. Check the first chapter for further instructions.

 How to Use It – Consume two cups a day.

145. IVY GOURD STEMS AND LEAVES (COOKED OR RAW) (COCCINIA INDICA)

 Medicinal Properties – There are a few active ingredients found in the Ivy gourd – amyran, taraxerone, taxerol, glycoside cucurbitacin B, and lupeol.

 Fun Fact – Ivy gourd has been used to treat constipation, wounds, and gonorrhea.

Why Will It Help – Because of its aforementioned active ingredients, it can destroy the free radicals within the body and can control the blood sugar levels.

 How to Make It

Ingredients – A few ivy gourd stems or leaves.

Instructions – Depending on your preferences, you can either add them to stews, soups, or salads (since they can be eaten raw and cooked).

 How to Use It – Add small amounts to your food a few times a week for up to 6 weeks for optimal results.

146. FIG LEAF INFUSION (FICUS CARICA)

 Medicinal Properties – It contains antiviral, antifungal, antidiabetes, antibacterial, antioxidant, and anti-cancer benefits.

 Fun Fact – The fig tree is native to the Mediterranean. Fig leaf sap is toxic to dogs.

 Why Will It Help – It is believed to assist glucose levels in the body, though its active component is still unknown.

 How to Make It

Ingredients – A handful of fresh fig leaves and a cup of water.

Instructions – Put the leaves on a baking sheet and bake them for 30 minutes. Then, crush them and proceed to make the infusion as per the instructions in the first chapter.

 How to Use It – 35 fig leaves equal 20 tea bags – consume a cup daily.

147. BITTER MELON DRIED FRUIT OR TEA (MOMORDICA CHARANTIA)

 Medicinal Properties – It contains many powerful antioxidants, including epicatechin, chlorogenic acid, gallic acid, and catechin.

 Fun Fact – The bitter taste of the bitter melon comes from a compound called cucurbitacin, which is present in members of the cucumber family to deter herbivores.

 Why Will It Help – The abovementioned antioxidants can protect the body from many diseases, including heart disease, cancer, and diabetes.

 How to Make It
Ingredients – 3-4 slices of fresh or dried bitter melon, and 1 cup of water, some honey (optional).

Instructions – Bring the water to a boil and then add the slices. Leave it to sit for a few minutes, and then strain. Add some honey if needed.

 How to Use It – Consume a cup a day while it is hot.

148. GURMAR POWDERED LEAVES (GYMNEMA SYLVESTRE)

 Medicinal Properties – It contains flavonols, saponins, gurmarin, and gymnemic acid IV (which has antihyperglycemic effects).

 Fun Fact – The leaves have been used in Ayurvedic medicine to treat constipation, cough, and allergies.

Why Will It Help – The compound gymnemic acid IV, when consumed orally along with diabetes medication, can reduce blood sugar in people who are dealing with diabetes type 1 or 2.

How to Make It

Ingredients – 1 teaspoon of powdered Gunmar leaves and 1 glass of water.

Instructions – Add the powdered Gunmar leaves to the glass of water and stir.

How to Use It – Consume one glass half an hour after lunch and dinner.

149. HOLY BASIL (OCIMUM TENUIFLORUM)

Medicinal Properties – This herb contains anti-inflammatory, antibacterial, antiviral, and hypoglycaemic properties.

Fun Fact – Some people chew fresh tulsi leaves every day to get the benefits from them.

Why Will It Help – If you have prediabetes or type 2 diabetes, all parts of the holy basil plant can help reduce your blood sugar levels. Animal and human studies have shown that holy basil can help prevent symptoms of diabetes, such as hyperinsulinemia, excess insulin in the blood, and weight gain.

How to Make It

Ingredients – A few leaves of holy basil and a cup of water.

Instructions – Boil the water and add the leaves to it. Let it sit for a few minutes.

How to Use It – Consume a cup every day.

150. MILK THISTLE EXTRACT (SILYBUM MARIANUM)

 Medicinal Properties – This plant provides anti-inflammatory, antioxidant, and blood sugar-lowering properties.

 Fun Fact – Historically, the milk thistle is native to Europe but has been introduced to Americans by early colonists.

Why will it help? – One of the active ingredients in this plant that has antioxidant properties is called silymarin. It is believed to assist the condition of people dealing with diabetes.

 How to Make It
Ingredients – 1 teaspoon or 1 tablespoon of milk thistle seeds, some water.

Instructions – Grind the seeds and add them to the pot of boiling water. Continue making the recipe as per the instructions in Chapter 1.

 How to Use It – Consume a cup a day.

151. FENUGREEK SEED (SOAKED, SPROUTED) (TRIGONELLA FOENUM-GRAECUM)

 Medicinal Properties – The fenugreek seeds are high in soluble fiber, which ultimately slows down digestion and controls blood sugar levels.

 Fun Fact – Another incredible plant that is native to the Mediterranean.

 Why Will It Help – Certain studies have shown that consuming fenugreek seeds twice a day before meals for three months can considerably decrease fasting blood glucose levels in people with diabetes.

How to Make It

Ingredients – 2 ½ teaspoons of fenugreek seeds and one glass of water.

Instructions – Heat the water (don't boil it) and add the fenugreek seeds to it. Leave it overnight.

How to Use It – Consume on an empty stomach first thing in the morning.

152. NOPAL LEAVES (OPUNTIA FOCUS-INDICA)

Medicinal Properties – It contains antiviral and anti-inflammatory properties.

Fun Fact – These leaves are an excellent source of magnesium, calcium, and Vitamin C.

Why Will It Help – Nopal leaves contain fiber, which is beneficial for managing diabetes. These can be a part of your high-fiber diet and ultimately lead to lowered blood sugar levels, reduced insulin levels, and improved fat compound levels (lipids) in the blood.

How to Make It

Ingredients – 3.5 oz of nopal leaves.

Instructions – Cook the leaves and add them as a garnish to your food.

How to Use It – Consume the leaves regularly – and incorporate them into your dietary plan.

153. CACTUS PINEAPPLE ORANGE JUICE

 Medicinal Properties – This drink will reduce high blood pressure and cholesterol levels and provide anti-inflammatory effects. It is filled with Vitamins A, C, and K, and also calcium, sodium, potassium, magnesium, phosphorous, etc.

 Fun Fact – This juice is believed to reduce the symptoms of alcohol hangover.

 Why Will It Help – Because it is a healthy, diabetic-friendly drink that contains the aforementioned vitamins and minerals.

 How to Make It
Ingredients – 1 cup of chopped fresh nopal leaves, 1 cucumber, 2 cups of chopped pineapple, 1 orange, and 1 cup of water.

Instructions – Peel the cucumber and cut it into pieces. Then, add it to a blender along with the other ingredients. Blend until smooth (for about 5 minutes until you get a thick juice).

 How to Use It – Consume one glass daily.

154. GYMNEMA TINCTURE (GYMNEMA SYLVESTRE)

 Medicinal Properties – Providing diuretic, astringent, antidiabetic, and hypoglycemic properties, it is an herb you should not overlook.

 Fun Fact – It has the ability to abolish the taste of sugar completely.

 Why Will It Help – Due to its anti-diabetic properties mentioned above, it controls the blood sugar levels of people who are dealing with diabetes.

How to Make It

Ingredients – A handful of the gymnema leaves, enough alcohol to cover them.

Instructions – Add the ingredients to a glass jar and continue making the tincture as per the instructions in the first chapter.

How to Use It – Maximum of ½ teaspoon directly on the tongue every 3 hours.

155. HERBAL BLOOD SUGAR BALANCE RECIPE

Medicinal Properties – This powerful mixture can help support blood sugar balance. It provides antibacterial, antioxidant, anti-inflammatory, antifungal, and antiviral properties.

Fun Fact – Many people have been using apple cider vinegar to control their blood sugar levels.

Why Will It Help – Because it will balance your blood sugar levels, thus balancing so many other functions – energy, weight, hormones, mood, and the health of the kidneys, eyes, heart, and more!

How to Make It

Ingredients – Some apple cider vinegar, 2-3 cinnamon sticks, ½ cup of tulsi parts.

Instructions – Place the cinnamon and tulsi in a glass jar and cover with ACV to the top. Secure the jar and leave it for 2 weeks in a cool and dark place. Then, strain the herbs and keep the liquid in a glass jar.

How to Use It – Consume 1-2 teaspoons of it, diluted in water, before meals. Use a straw when drinking it so the ACV does not destroy your teeth' enamel (due to the acidity).

156. CURRY LEAVES MIXTURE (MURRAYA KOENIGII)

 Medicinal Properties – Curry leaves are known all over the world as the best natural antioxidant. They also contain anti-inflammatory and antimicrobial properties.

 Fun Fact – The earliest recorded curry leaves recipe dates back to 1747.

 Why Will It Help – Because of their antioxidant properties, they can increase glucose absorption by cells.

 How to Make It

Ingredients – 8-9 curry leaves, 1 stick of cinnamon, a small piece of ginger, a teaspoon of fenugreek seeds, 2-3 glasses of water.

Instructions – Add all the ingredients to a pot and boil them on medium heat until only half of the mixture is left.

 How to Use It – Consume the entire portion in two equal parts.

157. JAMUN SEEDS (SYZYGIUM CUMINI)

 Medicinal Properties – Jamun seeds contain anti-inflammatory, diuretic, and antioxidant properties. Also, some bioactive compounds (flavonoids, phenols, saponins, terpenoids, and glycosides) stimulate insulin production, and to top it all off, they contain fiber and many micronutrients.

Fun Fact – The Jamun seeds are an excellent source of iron!

 Why Will It Help – Because the jamun seeds contain active compounds, which, along with the fiber, can help lower blood sugar levels by improving glucose utilization and enhancing insulin sensitivity.

 How to Make It

Ingredients – 20/25 jamun seeds.

Instructions – Completely dry the seeds. Blend the seeds until you create a powder. Mash them properly and store them in a jar.

 How to Use It – Take a tablespoon of the powder twice a day.

158. AMLA JUICE (PHYLLANTHUS EMBLICA)

 Medicinal Properties – Amlas are a powerhouse when it comes to antioxidants. They are the best choice for combating high sugar levels in the body.

 Fun Fact – Due to its high Vitamin C content, it is used to boost overall immunity.

 Why Will It Help – Because the amla can control the pancreatitis, thus helping the proper insulin production in the body. It increases the body's response to insulin and controls high blood sugar levels.

 How to Make It

Ingredients – 2 amlas and one glass of water.
Instructions – Grind the amlas and add the water. Mix well.

 How to Use It – – If necessary, add a pinch of salt to the mixture and drink the juice.

THE ROLE OF DIET IN KEEPING YOUR BLOOD SUGAR LEVELS IN-CHECK

Let's be honest – many factors contribute to checking your blood sugar levels. Whether you are a pre-diabetic or dealing with diabetes, you need to understand that three main factors contribute to your overall health and management of this condition. They are – physical activity, weight management, and healthy eating.

The role of a good diet can contribute a lot more than you think to your overall health. Sticking to a healthy consumption plan with foods filled with nutrients can help your body use insulin more efficiently. If you have diabetes, consuming healthy foods can help you:

- Maintain a healthy weight
- Prevent the development of diabetes complications
- Better management of your blood glucose levels
- Maintain a healthy blood pressure level
- Maintain overall good health

Some foods are recommended – so when you start building up your dietary plan, make the calories count! Here is what you need to choose:
- Healthy carbs include legumes, vegetables, fruits, whole grains, and low-fat dairy products.
- Fiber foods – legumes, nuts, fruits, vegetables, and whole grains.
- Fish – such as salmon, mackerel, tuna, and sardines.
- Good fats include olive oil, peanut oil, avocados, and nuts. Remember not to overdo it here, as all fats are very high in calories.

Avoid sodium, trans fats, saturated fats, and cholesterol-filled foods – such as sausages, bacon, butter, beef, hot dogs, coconut oil, baked goods, margarine, animal protein, egg yolks, and processed snacks.

After considering all of this, you will soon learn that there is an easy and healthy way to boost your immune system and keep your blood sugar levels in check. There is no need to panic – all you need to do is stick to the instructions and medication given to you by your health provider and try these herbal recipes.

I suggest giving all of them a go – and stick to the ones you prefer the most!

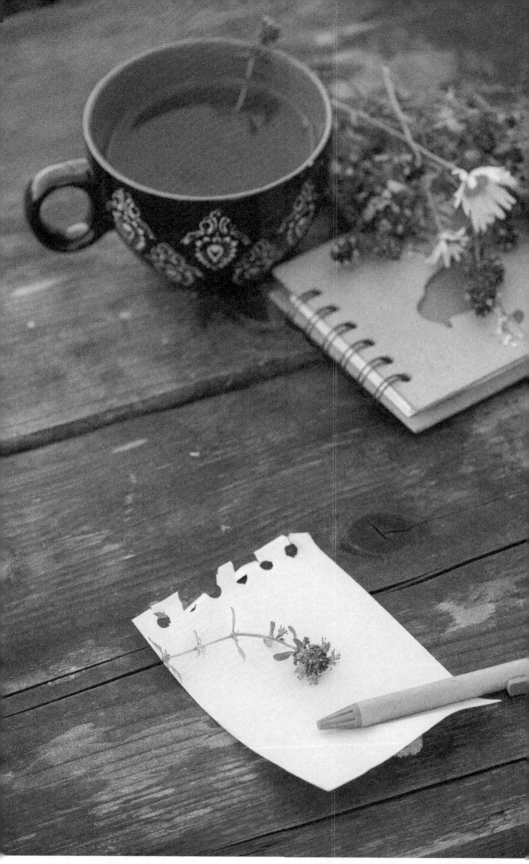

CONCLUSION

In a world filled with people constantly struggling to maintain their overall health, be the one who is always a few steps ahead. Giving a chance for alternative medicine to shine through your kitchen and into your life is the perfect way to keep your optimal health!

After everything you have learned so far, how do you feel about giving these recipes a go?

Remember, we may have come to the end of this chapter together, but it is not the end of our journey. As you walk through this book time and time again, you will enjoy the wide range of herbal medicine, each time uncovering something new and exciting. Learning the power plants have to improve our overall well-being is thrilling – and knowing the ancient wisdom by heart is an absolute joy.

The herbal remedies are cost-effective, accessible, and effective overall. Whether you are a seasoned herbal enthusiast or someone who is just getting started, you have probably realized the healing potential of some herbs (some you might have even used by now). Learning how to make some wonders at home can lead to a special connection.

One of the most remarkable aspects of herbal medicine is its ability to assist with various health issues, from minor ones to more serious ones. When reading this book, you have discovered both and learned about herbs that can soothe your entire body, mind, and even spirit. With the perfect guide from the beginning of this book, you can tailor the remedies to fit your needs. Implement a little bit of safety when practicing herbal medicine at home. As I have mentioned many times before, from some of the most potent ingredients, try them in extra small doses before going to bigger ones. Or, talk to your health provider to ensure they will not interfere with any medication you might be taking. Also, correctly identify the ingredient before using it.

As this final chapter ends, you can stop for a minute and reflect on everything you have learned. Tapping into the rich plethora of herbal remedies and exploring your options has never been easier. Through the help of this book, you have discovered how to create creams, tinctures, teas, and juices and embrace their powers. These are not new recipes – but rather ancient ones that have stood the test of time. They have been a trusted ally to the health journey of many generations before you – and will hopefully still be present for many generations to come!

While you are on your way to achieving your health goals, don't forget to look back – remind yourself of a recipe each time you feel like you need some support. After all, that is what this book is about. Also, don't forget to look ahead too! The second part of my book is in the making and will cover an entirely new plethora of herbal remedies, as well as their medicinal benefits. So be on the lookout for it – it should come out sooner than you expect!

As I am saying goodbye to you for now, I urge you to always look after yourself – and incorporate the herbal wisdom from this book in all aspects of your life. Create a healthier, happier, and more joyful you! Fill your future with bliss and a positive attitude, add the ingredients from the recipes, and enjoy life to the fullest!

I would love to hear your feedback on my book – show your support by leaving a review!

REFERENCES

CHAPTER ONE: HOW TO MAKE NATURAL REMEDIES AT HOME (TEAS, TINCTURES, SALVES, ETC), SAFETY WARNINGS

22 Easy Herbal Recipes For Teas, Tinctures, An More. Nourished Kitchen. https://nourishedkitchen.com/herbalism/#:~:text=You%20make%20them%20by%20macerating,from%20oil%2Dbased%20extraction%20methods

Me icinal Herbs. The Herb Garden https://theherbgarden.ie/using-herbs/medicinal-herbs/

James. (23 November 2021). *How To Make Herbal Reme ies At Home.* Totally Wild UK. https://totallywilduk.co.uk/2021/11/23/how-to-make-herbal-remedies-at-home/

Dana. (5 September 2019). *10 Essential Tools Every Herbalist Nee s.* Rustic Farm Life. https://www.rusticfarmlife.com/essential-tools-every-herbalist-needs/

Mason. (1 February 2018). *Must-Have Tools For Herbalists.* Mountain Rose Herbs. https://blog.mountainroseherbs.com/tools-for-herbalists

Herbal Me icine. Johns Hopkins Medicine. https://www.hopkinsmedicine.org/health/wellness-and-prevention/herbal-medicine

*5 Steps To Take Herbal Me*icine Safely.* Jennifer Raye Medicine And Movement. https://jenniferraye.com/herbal-safety/

CHAPTER TWO: REMEDIES FOR DIGESTIVE (GUT) HEALTH

RealGingerTeaForGutHealth. FairfieldNutrition. https://fairfieldnutrition.com. au/2020/03/28/ginger-tea-recipe-for-gut-health/#:~:text=Real%20 Ginger%20Tea%20for%20Gut%20Health&text=Drinking%20 ginger%20tea%20regularly%20may,associated%20with%20chronic%20 gut%20inflammation

(20 February 2023). *Best Digestive Tea Recipe.* Good For Baddie. https:// goodfoodbaddie.com/best-digestive-tea-recipe/

Villanueva, L. *How To Make Favorite Healthy Digestion Peppermint Tea Recipe.* Eat Your Nutrition. https://recipes.eatyournutrition.com/ teas-for-healthy-digestion/

Groves, Noel, M. *Herbal Tea Blen*s For Goo* Gut Health.* Hachette Book Group. https://www.hachettebookgroup.com/storey/ herbal-tea-gut-health/?lens=storey

Heidi. (21 November 2022). *Bitter, Aromatic, An* Demulcent Herbs For Digestion + 3 Recipes.* Mountain Rose Herbs. https://blog.mountainroseherbs. com/herbs-healthy-digestion-recipes

(26 August 2013). *Psyllium See*s Husk – A Natural Reme*y For IBS.* Charlestown Medical Centre. https://www.charlestownmedicalcentre.ie/our-blog/ psyllium-seeds-husk-a-natural-remedy-for-ibs

White, A. (28 February 2019). *Can Aloe Vera Juice Treat IBS?* Healthline. https:// www.healthline.com/health/digestive-health/aloe-vera-juice-for-ibs

Bolen, B. (5 August 2022). *The Use Of Triphala In Treating IBS.* Very Well Health. https:// www.verywellhealth.com/triphala-for-stomach-problems-and-ibs-1944993

Vasu, D. (13 March 2023). *Triphala – Benefits, Nutrition, An Recipes.* Healthify Me. https://www.healthifyme.com/blog/triphala/#Best_Ways_to_Consume_Triphala

Metropulos, M. (23 January 2018). *Best Teas To Drink For IBS.* Medical News Today. https://www.medicalnewstoday.com/articles/320705#:~:text=Eating%20turmeric%20has%20relatively%20little,a%20piece%20of%20turmeric%20root

Anti-Inflammatory Turmeric Tea Recipe (Golen Milk). Elisabeth Rider. https://www.elizabethrider.com/how-to-make-golden-milk-recipe/

Dessinger, H. *4 Artichoke Leaf Benefits + How To Use It.* Mommypotamus. https://mommypotamus.com/artichoke-leaf-benefits/

Mangaluru, B. (22 November 2022). *Natural Solution. Cranberry Juice Can Help Prevent H.Pylori Bacterial Infection, Strengthen Gut Health.* The Hindu Business Line. https://www.thehindubusinessline.com/news/science/cranberry-juice-can-help-prevent-h-pylori-bacterial-infection-strengthen-gut-health/article66164534.ece

(3 August 2023). *Homemae Cranberry Juice.* Taste Of Home. https://www.tasteofhome.com/recipes/homemade-cranberry-juice/

Singh, A. (28 November 2020). *Lemongrass Oil Uses, Benefits, An How to Make It At Home.* Vitsupp. https://www.vitsupp.com/lemongrass-oil/

Naser, S. (7 July 2023). *11 Home Remeies To Get Ri Of Helicobacter Pylori Infection.* Stylecraze. https://www.stylecraze.com/articles/helicobacter-pylori-natural-treatment/#GreenTea

Bodhare, A. (27 June 2023). *Natural Home Remeies For Stomach Ulcers.* PharmEasy. https://pharmeasy.in/blog/home-remedies-for-stomach-ulcers/

Swasthi. (24 June 2023). *Amla Juice Recipe (Gooseberry Juice Shots).* Indian Healthy Recipes. https://www.indianhealthyrecipes.com/amla-juice-with-manuka-honey-indian-gooseberry/

Anupama. (21 February 2016). *Duo⬦enal An⬦ Gastric Ulcer Ayurve⬦ic Me⬦icines An⬦ Dosages.* Bimbima. https://www.bimbima.com/ayurveda/duodenal-and-gastric-ulcer-ayurvedic-medicines-and-dosages/119/

CHAPTER THREE: REMEDIES FOR SKIN HEALTH

Herbs, G. (15 May 2022). *The 9 Best Herbs To Support Healthy, Glowing Skin From The Insi⬦e Out.* Gaia Herbs. https://www.gaiaherbs.com/blogs/seeds-of-knowledge/the-7-best-herbal-supplements-for-healthy-glowing-skin-from-the-inside-out

Shah, N. (8 October 2021). *Have You Trie⬦ Using Neem For Acne? Here Are 6 Effective Ways To Do So.* Be Beautiful. https://www.bebeautiful.in/all-things-skin/skin-concerns/neem-for-acne#neem-and-sandalwood-face-pack

Bose, S. (17 June 2021). *Herbs For Acne: Benefits An⬦ How To Use Them.* Be Beautiful. https://www.bebeautiful.in/all-things-skin/skin-concerns/herbs-for-acne

(20 November 2019). *How To Make The Most Soothing Oatmeal Bath Ever.* Greatist. https://greatist.com/eczema/oatmeal-bath-for-eczema

(12 March 2022). *Easy Homema⬦e Eczema Cream With Aloe Vera.* Fivespot Green Living. https://www.fivespotgreenliving.com/homemade-eczema-cream-with-aloe-vera/

Delzell, E. (21 June 2020). *Get The Facts: Turmeric.* Natural Eczema Association. https://nationaleczema.org/blog/get-the-facts-turmeric/

Alabata, T. (23 Janruary 2019). *DIY Gentle Chamomile Calen⬦ula Healing Balm For Face An⬦ Scalp Eczema.* Atopic Dermatitis. https://atopicdermatitis.net/living/diy-eczema-healing-balm

Carter, E. (16 April 2023). *5 Best Essential Oils For Rosacea.* Essential Oil Haven. https://www.essentialoilhaven.com/essential-oils-for-rosacea/

Aryal, O. (30 September 2020). *Essential Oils For Rosacea: What To Include In Your Skincare Routine.* Motherhood Community. https://motherhoodcommunity. com/essential-oils-for-rosacea/#how-to-use-essential-oils-for-rosacea

15 Interesting And Effective Treatments For Rosacea. Rhoose Point Remedies. https://rhoosepointremedies.com/15-interesting-and-effective-treatements-for-rosacea/#Green-Tea-Skin-Soak

Hamdani, S. (28 September 2021). *Ayurvedic Treatment For Dandruff: 5 Natural Remedies That Work.* Be Beautiful. https://www.bebeautiful. in/all-things-hair/hair-concerns/ayurvedic-treatment-for-dandruff

Rosemary Oil And Its Effects On Dandruff. Head & Shoulders. https://www. headandshoulders.co.in/en-in/healthy-hair-and-scalp/dandruff/dandruff-home-remedies/rosemary-oil-for-dandruff

Glenn, A. (14 December 2015). *Coltsfoot Rinse – A Natural Remedy For Dandruff.* Naturally Curly. https://www.naturallycurly.com/curlreading/ingredients/coltsfoot-tussilago-rinse-for-hair#

Madison, N. (7 September 2023). *How Effective Is Flaxseed Oil For Acne?* The Health Board. https://www.thehealthboard.com/how-effective-is-flaxseed-oil-for-acne.htm

Shamsher, S. *Flaxseeds And Acne.* Dr. Health Clinic. https://www. drhealthclinic.com/flaxseeds-and-acne/

What Is Purslane Tea? Brewed Leaf Love. https://brewedleaflove.com/what-is-purslane-tea/

Tabassum, N., Hamdani, M. (June 2014). *Plants Used To Treat Skin Diseases.* National Center For Biotechnology Information. https://www.ncbi. nlm.nih.gov/pmc/articles/PMC3931201/

Patnaik, V. (7 July 2023). *Purslane Benefits An♦ Si♦e Effects: A Comprehensive Gui♦e.* Stylecraze. https://www.stylecraze.com/articles/purslane-benefits/

Barode, S. (11 September 2023). *Ashokarishta: Uses, Benefits, Si♦e Effects, Precautions, & More!* PharmEasy. https://pharmeasy.in/blog/ayurveda-uses-benefits-side-effects-of-ashokarishta/

(5 August 2020). *Benefits Of Ashoka Tree An♦ Its Si♦e Effects.* Lybrate. https://www.lybrate.com/topic/ashoka-tree-uses-benefits-and-side-effects

Basu, S. (29 July 2022). *Bhringaraj: Benefits For Hair, Uses, Dosage, Formulations, An♦ Si♦e Effects.* Netmeds.com. https://www.netmeds.com/health-library/post/bhringaraj-benefits-for-hair-uses-dosage-formulations-and-side-effects

Pal, Y., Wal, A., Wal, P., Saraswat, N., Pal, S. (6 July 2020). *Preparation & Assessment Of Poly-Herbal Anti-Dan♦ruff Formulation.* Open Dermatology Journal. https://opendermatologyjournal.com/VOLUME/14/PAGE/22/FULLTEXT/

Sylvia. (29 July 2018). *Facts An♦ Benefits Of Devil's Horsewhip (Chaff Flower).* Health Benefits Times. https://www.healthbenefitstimes.com/devils-horsewhip/

Bantilan, C. (24 October 2019). *What Is Oregon Grape? Uses An♦ Si♦e Effects.* Healthline. https://www.healthline.com/nutrition/oregon-grape

The Skin Benefits Of Cannabis Sativa See♦ Oil. Kiehls. https://www.kiehls.com/skincare-advice/cannabis.html

Surprising Benefits Of Camphor: Camphor Skin Benefits For Whitening An♦ Ra♦iance. Vicco Labs. https://viccolabs.com/blogs/vicco-laboratories/surprising-benefits-of-camphor-camphor-skin-benefits-for-whitening-and-radiance

CHAPTER FOUR: REMEDIES FOR RESPIRATORY HEALTH

Welch, S. (30 November 2021). *9 Herbs To Relieve Cola Ana Flu Symptoms.* Farm And Dairy. https://www.farmanddairy.com/top-stories/9-herbs-to-relieve-cold-and-flu-symptoms/695280.html

Baillie,L.(1October2020).*6HelpfulHerbsForAllergySufferers.*A.Vogel.https://www.avogel.co.uk/health/allergic-rhinitis/6-helpful-herbs-for-allergy-sufferers/

(10 July 2018). *6 Herbal Remeaies For Allergic Rhinitis.* Sinus & Allergy Wellness Clinic. https://www.sinusandallergywellnesscenter.com/blog/allergic-rhinitis-6-herbal-remedies-to-try-sinus-allergy-wellness-clinic

(2 January 2018). *7 Effective Home Remeaies To Cure Asthma.* Times Of India. https://recipes.timesofindia.com/articles/health/7-effective-home-remedies-to-cure-asthma/photostory/62337043.cms

(23 October 2019). *Black Seea Oil For Asthma + 3 Practical Ways To Use It.* Nature's Blends. https://www.naturesblends.com/blogs/news/black-seed-oil-for-asthma

Anupama. (30 January 2014). *Asthma Weea Or Tawa-Tawa (Euphorbia Hirta) Tea.* Bimbima. https://www.bimbima.com/recipes/asthma-weed-or-tawa-tawa-euphorbia-hirta-tea/2302/

Price,A.(29August2018).*Top5EssentialOilsForAsthmaSymptoms.*Dr.Axe.https://draxe.com/essential-oils/essential-oils-for-asthma-symptoms/#:~:text=Want%20to%20know%20the%20best,Then%20take%20deep%2C%20diaphragmatic%20breaths

(24 February 2020). *Allergy Fighting Tea Recipe.* Grow Create Sip. https://www.growcreatesip.com/blog/allergy-fighting-tea-recipe

Johnson, L. (10 March 2020). *How To Make Herbal Tea For Allergies + Recipes.* Hello You. https://helloglow.co/herbal-tea-for-allergies/

Gibson, B. (29 March 2023). *Herbal Allergy Tea Recipe For Relief.* The Homestead Challenge. https://thehomesteadchallenge.com/herbal-allergy-tea-recipe/

Stewart, M. (22 January 2019). *Anti Allergy Tea.* Martha Stewart. https://www.marthastewart.com/1155942/anti-allergy-tea

Anti-Allergy Tea. Dr. Kara Fitzgerald. https://www.drkarafitzgerald.com/recipe/anti-allergy-tea/

Cumberland, J. (3 October 2022). *9 Natural Remedies For Bronchitis Treatment.* eMediHealth. https://www.emedihealth.com/respiratory-health/lung-diseases/natural-remedies-bronchitis

Bharat, D. (21 June 2021). *Ayurveda For Bronchitis: Proven Natural Remedies To Pacify Lung Inflammation And Breathe Easy.* Netmeds.com. https://www.netmeds.com/health-library/post/ayurveda-for-bronchitis-proven-natural-remedies-to-pacify-lung-inflammation-and-breathe-easy

Binu, S. (26 April 2021). *Tulsi Tea: 5 Incredible Health Reasons To Include This Energising Beverage In Your Regimen.* Netmeds.com. https://www.netmeds.com/health-library/post/tulsi-tea-5-incredible-health-reasons-to-include-this-energising-beverage-in-your-regimen?utm_source=Blog-Post&utm_medium=Post&utm_campaign=NMSBlogPost

(4 November 2020). *Body Care Recipe: Lung & Chest Rub.* The Herb Shoppe PDX. https://theherbshoppepdx.com/blogs/blog/body-care-recipe-lung-chest-rub

Grieve, K. (February 2012). *How To Make Thyme Tea For Colds And Coughs.* Larder Love. https://larderlove.com/thyme-tea-for-colds-and-caughs/

Eco-Age.(21 January 2019). *6 Gar enHerbsForFluSeason.* Eco-Age.https://eco-age.
com/resources/6-garden-herbs-flu-season/#:~:text=Also%2C%20
Rosemary%20is%20another%20great,breathe%20in%20the%20rising%20
steam

Academy, H. (13 January 2014). *8 Supportive Herbs For Col s
An Flu.* The Herbal Academy. https://theherbalacademy.
com/8-herbal-home-remedies-for-colds-and-flu/

Kring, L. (14 September 2021). *Make Soothing Herbal Tea For Coughs, Col s,
An The Flu.* Gardener's Path. https://gardenerspath.com/plants/
herbs/herbal-tea/

Maine.gov. *Fun Bee an Honey Facts.* https://www.maine.gov/dacf/php/
integrated_pest_management/school-ipm-curricula/elementary/
documents/FunBeeFacts.pdf

National Institute of Health (2014) Cinnamon: A Multifaceted Medicinal
Plant https://www.ncbi.nlm.nih.gov/pmc/articles/PMC4003790

CHAPTER FIVE: REMEDIES FOR CARDIOVASCULAR HEALTH

Chauhan,M.(29 April 2019). *HomeReme iesforBlocke Arteries.* PlanetAyurveda.https://
www.planetayurveda.com/library/home-remedies-for-blocked-arteries/

(30 January 2019). *OnlyAGlassOfThisJuiceWillRemoveClogge ArteriesAn ControlBloo
Pressure.* Fars News. https://www.farsnews.ir/en/news/13971110000376/
Only-a-Glass-f-This-Jice-will-Remve-Clgged-Areries-And-Cnrl-Bld

Artery Blockage, Herbs, An Home Reme ies. Planet Ayurveda. https://www.
planetayurveda.com/artery-blockage-herbs-and-home-remedies/

Chauhan, M. (14 February 2019). *Ayurve ic Treatment Of Abnormal Heart
Rhythms (Arrythmia).* Planet Ayurveda. https://www.planetayurveda.
com/library/abnormal-heart-rhythms/

Marshall, K. (18 August 2021). *Motherwort Tincture Recipe.* Home Garden Joy. https://homegardenjoy.com/site/2021/08/motherwort-tincture-recipe.html

Joybilee Farm. *How To Make The Most Effective Hawthorn Berry Syrup Heart Tonic.* Joybilee Farm. https://joybileefarm.com/hawthorn-syrup-heart-tonic/

Lanae, T. *Heart Tea Recipe For Arrhythmia And Better Circulation – Quick & Easy!!! (Must See).* YouTube. https://www.youtube.com/watch?v=XByNHS8BqZk

Reis, M. (May 2022). *13 Home Remedies For High Blood Pressure.* Tua Saude. https://www.tuasaude.com/en/natural-remedies-for-high-blood-pressure/

Publishing, S. *Sneak Peek: Rosemary Gladstar's Herbal Healing For Men.* Scribd. https://www.scribd.com/document/347723976/Sneak-Peek-Rosemary-Gladstar-s-Herbal-Healing-for-Men

Bantilan, C. (12 December 2019). *5 Emerging Benefits And Uses Of Yarrow Tea.* Healthline. https://www.healthline.com/nutrition/yarrow-tea

CHAPTER SIX: REMEDIES FOR IMMUNE HEALTH

Bedosky, L. (1 December 2022). *7 Herbs And Spices That May Help Boost Immunity Naturally.* Everyday Health. https://www.everydayhealth.com/diet-nutrition/herbs-and-spices-that-may-help-boost-immunity-naturally/

Ruggeri, C. (12 June 2019). *Olive Leaf Extract Benefits For Cardiovascular Health And Brain Function.* Dr. Axe. https://draxe.com/nutrition/olive-leaf-benefits/

Adaptogens: 75+ Herbal Recipes And Elixirs To Improve Your Skin, Mood, Energy, Focus, And More. Chapter 6 – Recipes To Improve Your Immune Function. Doctor Lib. https://doctorlib.info/herbal/adaptogens/6.html

Jessicka. (8 January 2022). *Adaptogenic Chai Tea Recipe With Astragalus.* Mountain Rose Herbs. https://blog.mountainroseherbs.com/ astragalus-chai-immune-support-recipe

Dog, T. (25 August 2021). *How To Make Elderberry Syrup For Immune System Suport.* Mountain Rose Herbs. https://blog.mountainroseherbs.com/ elderberry-syrup-recipe

(18 September 2023). *4 Best Teas For Liver Detox & Repair Liver Functions.* Vahdam. https://www.vahdam.com/blogs/tea-us/4-best-teas-for-liver-detox-repair-liver-functions

Top Three Immune Boosting Elderberry Tonic Recipes. Seedmart. https://seedmart. com.au/top-three-immune-boosting-elderberry-tonic-recipes/

Shahani, S. (20 May 2020). *8 Herbal Tea Recipes To Boost Your Immune System.* Conde Nast Traveller. https://www.cntraveller.in/story/8-herbal-tea-recipes-to-boost-your-immune-system-turmeric-haldi-ginger-tulsi/

CHAPTER SEVEN: REMEDIES FOR URINARY TRACT SYSTEM

Oregon Grape. Wild Foods & Medicines. https://wildfoodsandmedicines. com/oregon-grape/

Adamant, A. (3 May 2018). *How To Make Dandelion Tincture.* Practical Self Reliance. https://practicalselfreliance.com/dandelion-tincture/

Parvanova, I. *Cranberry Tea For Healthy Urinary Tract.* Bonapeti. https:// bonapeti.com/recipes/r-190618-Cranberry_Tea_for_Healthy_ Urinary_Tract

Devon. *Urinary Herbs: Uva-Ursi For Good Bladder Health & Relief.* Nitty Gritty Life. https://nittygrittylife.com/uva-ursi-bladder-health/

Zanin, T. (March 2022). *Parsley Tea For Urinary Tract Infection (UTI): 3 Best Recipes.* Tua Saude. https://www.tuasaude.com/en/parsley-tea-to-treat-a-urinary-tract-infection/

Reis, M. (December 2022). *Best Herbs For UTI Treatment: 6 Tea Recipes.* Tua Saude. https://www.tuasaude.com/en/teas-for-uti/

Nelson, C. *Home Remedies.* Women's Health Specialists. https://www.womenshealthspecialists.org/self-help/home-remedies/

Ganguly, S. (27 February 2019). *Remedies For Cloudy Urine?* Glossy Polish. https://glossypolish.com/remedies-cloudy-urine/

Kukreja, K. (7 July 2023). *10 Effective Home Remedies To Help With Cloudy Urine.* Stylecraze. https://www.stylecraze.com/articles/effective-home-remedies-to-treat-cloudy-urine/#home-remedies-for-cloudy-urine

Mullein Tea Recipe. Edible Wild Food. https://www.ediblewildfood.com/mullein-tea.aspx

CHAPTER EIGHT: BONE, LIGAMENT, AND MUSCLE HEALTH

Mueller, J., Barcal, L. (21 January 2022). *How To Make Clove Oil.* WikiHow. https://www.wikihow.com/Make-Clove-Oil

Bell, A. (22 May 2020). *Camphor Oil: Types, Uses, And Products.* Medical News Today. https://www.medicalnewstoday.com/articles/camphor-oil

(12 November 2020). *How To Make Chamomile Oil At Home.* Blend It Raw Apothecary. https://blenditrawapothecary.in/blogs/body-care-recipes/how-to-make-chamomile-oil-at-home

(21 August 2022). *Health Benefits Of Cayenne Pepper.* WebMD. https://www.webmd.com/diet/health-benefits-cayenne-pepper

Dessinger, H. *Arnica Cream Recipe (Video Tutorial).* Mommypotamus. https://mommypotamus.com/arnica-cream/

Devil's Claw – Uses, Side Effects, And More. WebMD. https://www.webmd.com/vitamins/ai/ingredientmono-984/devils-claw

Marik, B. (13 November 2017). *DIY With Frankincense (Boswellia Serrata).* Banyan Botanicals. https://www.banyanbotanicals.com/info/blog-the-banyan-insight/details/diy-with-frankincense-boswellia-serrata/

Boswellia Serrata - Uses, Side Effects, And More. WebMD. https://www.webmd.com/vitamins/ai/ingredientmono-63/boswellia-serrata

Shoemaker, S. (4 October 2019). *How To Make Aloe Vera Gel.* Healthline. https://www.healthline.com/nutrition/how-to-make-aloe-vera-gel

Homemade Ginger Ointment For Quick Pain Relief. Natural Cures. YoutTube. https://www.youtube.com/watch?v=7xW7blqOZOw

Berry, J. (30 July 2019). *10 Healthful Turmeric Recipes For Arthritis.* Medical News Today. https://www.medicalnewstoday.com/articles/325902

(14 March 2011). *Make White Willow Bark Tea For Pain Relief.* Mother Earth Living. https://www.motherearthliving.com/health-and-wellness/make-white-willow-bark-tea-for-pain-relief/

Axe, J. (29 January 2023). *DIY Arthritis Ointment For Joint Pain.* Dr. Axe. https://draxe.com/beauty/diy-arthritis-ointment/

Cherney, K. (15 November 2022). *9 Herbs To Fight Arthritis Pain.* Healthline. https://www.healthline.com/health/osteoarthritis/herbs-arthritis-pain

(16 January 2021). Homemade Arnica Salve Recipe. Homesteading Family. https://homesteadingfamily.com/homemade-arnica-salve-recipe/

Rebecca. *Chamomile Flowers Bath Tea Recipe.* Indigo Herbs. https://www. indigo-herbs.co.uk/recipe/chamomile-flowers-bath-tea

3 Natural Pain Killers For Your Back Or Nect Pain. Saratoga Spine. https:// saratogaspine.com/3-natural-pain-killers-for-your-back-or-neck- pain/

Storozhuk, Y. (9 September 2021). *Cory♦alis For Pain Relief + Dosage, Si♦e Effects & Reviews.* SelfDecode. https://supplements.selfdecode.com/ blog/corydalis/

(6 August 2021). *Pain-Be-Gone Valerian Cor♦ial With Willow.* The Herbal Academy. https://theherbalacademy.com/valerian-cordial/

Minesh. (11 March 2022). *Herbs An♦ Spices That Help With Back Pain.* The Spine Clinic. https://spineclinics.co.uk/herbs-for-back-pain/

(2022). *Five Herbs That Can Naturally Heal Back Pain.* Premier Health Chiropractors. https://premierhealthmn. com/5-herbs-that-can-naturally-heal-back-pain/

Blankespoor, J. (25 September 2023). *The Healing Benefits Of Gotu Kola: An E♦ible An♦ Me♦icinal Herb.* Chestnut Herbs. https://chestnutherbs. com/the-healing-benefits-of-gotu-kola/

Gibson, J., Burson, J. (4 June 2023). How To Make Fenugreek Tea. WikiHow. https://www.wikihow.com/Make-Fenugreek-Tea

How To Make Rho♦iola Rosea Tincture. Wilder Land Botanicals. https://wilderlandbotanicals.com/blogs/herbal-recipes/ how-to-make-rhodiola-rosea-herbal-tincture

Sage Tincture Recipe. Herbalism Roots. https://herbalismroots.com/ sage-tincture-recipe/#:~:text=Chop%20the%20sage%20and%20 place,into%20a%20colored%20glass%20container

(July 2020). Exercise And Bone Health. OrthiInfo. https://orthoinfo.aaos.org/ en/staying-healthy/exercise-and-bone-health/#:~:text=Exercise%20 is%20important%20for%20building,more%20bone%20and%20 becoming%20denser

CHAPTER NINE: ANXIETY

Alice. (2 April 2020). *Warming Fresh Ginger Chamomile Tea*. Sugar Salted. https://www.sugarsalted.com/warming-fresh-ginger-chamomile-tea/

(10 September 2020). *Ayurve ir Milk Recipes*. Ayush. https://www. ayurvedasg.com/ayurvedic-milk-recipes/

Richards, L. (9 February 2023). 9 Herbs For Anxiety. Medical News Today. https:// www.medicalnewstoday.com/articles/herbs-for-anxiety#how-do-they-work

Webber, J. *Herbs For Happiness: Plants To Boost Your Moo*. Pukka Herbs. https://www.pukkaherbs.com/uk/en/wellbeing-articles/ herbs-for-happiness

Ratini, M. (5 April 2022). *Herbs, Vitamins, An Supplements Use To Enhance Moo*. WebMD. https://www.webmd.com/diet/features/ herbs-vitamins-and-supplements-used-to-enhance-mood

Kennedy, K. (5 August 2022). *How To Make Valerian Tea*. Everyday Health. https://www.everydayhealth.com/diet-nutrition/make-valerian-tea-how-prepare-brew-steep-this-herbal-tea/

Moran, S. (2 September 2022). *How To Make Lemon Balm Tea*. The View From Great Island. https://theviewfromgreatisland.com/ how-to-make-lemon-balm-tea/

Maca Adaptogen Blend For Stress. The Maca Team. https://www. themacateam.com/maca-adaptogen-blend-for-stress

Uniyal, P. (7 August 2022). *Herbs For Happiness: 7 Amazing Herbs To Increase Happy Hormones, Balance Emotions*. Hindustan Times. https://www.hindustantimes.com/lifestyle/health/herbs-for-happiness-7-amazing-herbs-to-increase-happy-hormones-balance-emotions-101659862197361.html

Six Simple Jatamansi Recipes. Amrutam. https://amrutam.co.in/blogs/amrutam-daily-lifestyle/six-simple-jatamansi-recipes#:~:text=Take%2025%20grams%20of%20Jatamansi,it%20for%2024%20%E2%80%93%2036%20hours

Ningthoujam, N. *Herbs For Happiness: Take The Ayurvedic Route To Boost Your Mood*. Health Shots. https://www.healthshots.com/mind/happiness-hacks/herbs-for-happiness-take-the-ayurvedic-route-to-boost-your-mood/

Adaptogens: 75+ Herbal Recipes And Elixirs To Improve Your Skin, Mood, Energy, Focus, And More. Chapter 4 – Recipes To Improve Your Mood. Doctor Lib. https://doctorlib.info/herbal/adaptogens/4.html

Sneak Peek: Rosemary Gladstar's Herbal Healing For Men. Scribd. https://www.scribd.com/document/347723976/Sneak-Peek-Rosemary-Gladstar-s-Herbal-Healing-for-Men

Dessinger, H. *Passionflower Tea Recipe*. Mommypotamus. https://mommypotamus.com/passionflower-tea-recipe/

(26 April 2016). *An Elixir For Sleep; Kava Kava*. Dr. Hannah Webb. http://www.drhannahwebb.com/read-all-posts/2016/4/24/an-elixir-for-sleep-and-anxiety

Williams, C. (2 March 2022). *11 Calming Diys To Help Reduce Worry And Anxiety*. Brit+Co. https://www.brit.co/diys-that-help-with-anxiety/

(30 November 2022). *5 Herbal Tea Recipes To Relieve Anxiety And Stress*. Better Sleep. https://www.bettersleep.com/blog/5-herbal-tea-recipe-to-relieve-anxiety-and-stress/

Aromatherapy Recipes For Anxiety. Aroma Web. https://www.aromaweb. com/recipes/anxiety-recipes-blends-with-essential-oils.php

CHAPTER TEN: DIABETES

Dessinger, H. *8 Benefits Of Milk Thistle + How To Use It.* Mommypotamus. https://mommypotamus.com/benefits-of-milk-thistle/

Bonneau, A. (14 July 2023*). How to make fig leaf tea with forage♦ fig leaves.* Zero Waste Chef. https://zerowastechef.com/2023/07/14/ make-fig-leaf-tea/

Riverwalk Nursery. Facebook. https://www.facebook.com/riverwalknursery/ posts/did-you-know-that-orchid-tree-leaves-are-beneficial-dont-believe-me-read-below-i/2130472787024362/

(15 January 2019). *Herbal An♦ Natural Therapies.* Diabetes.Co. https://www. diabetes.co.uk/Diabetes-herbal.html

(15 September 2018). *Gurmar For Diabetes: Why This "Sugar Destroying" Herb Shoul♦ Be Part Of Your Diabetes Diet.* NDTV. https://www.ndtv.com/ food/gurmar-for-diabetes-why-this-sugar-destroying-herb-should-be-part-of-your-diabetes-diet-1917019

(21 September 2018). *Tulsi Leaves For Diabetes: How To Use Holy Basil To Manage Bloo♦ Sugar Levels.* NDTV. https://www.ndtv.com/food/ tulsi-leaves-for-diabetes-how-to-use-holy-basil-to-manage-blood-sugar-levels-1919011

Milk Thistle – Uses, Si♦e Effects, An♦ More. WebMD. https://www.webmd.com/ vitamins/ai/ingredientmono-138/milk-thistle#:~:text=Diabetes.,levels%20 in%20people%20with%20diabetes

(8 August 2022). *How To Use Fenugreek See♦s For Diabetes?* FitterFly. https:// www.fitterfly.com/blog/how-to-use-fenugreek-seeds-for-diabetes/

Johnson, J. (28 April 2023). *7 Herbs An♦ Supplements For Type 2 Diabetes.* Medical News Today. https://www.medicalnewstoday.com/articles/317051

Brown, G. (19 March 2019). *Treating Diabetes With Herbal Me♦icine?* Healthline. https://www.healthline.com/diabetesmine/treating-diabetes-herbal-medicine

Swathi. (20 January 2013). *Cactus Pineapple Orange Juice/ Agua De Nopal, Pina Con Naranja: A Diabetic Frien♦ly Juice.* Zesty South Indian Kitchen. https://zestysouthindiankitchen.com/cactus-pineapple-orange-juice/

Gymnema Sylvestre. The Naturopathic Herbalist. https://thenaturopathicherbalist.com/herbs/g-h/gymnema-sylvestre/

(21 March 2023). *Herbal Bloo♦ Sugar Balance Recipe.* The Herbal Academy. https://theherbalacademy.com/blood-sugar-balance/

Chandrashekara, A. (21 April 2022). *Top 10 Natural Home Reme♦ies For Diabetes.* Breathe Well-Being. https://www.breathewellbeing.in/blog/top-10-natural-home-remedies-for-diabetes-high-low-sugar/

(13 April 2023). *Diabetes Diet: Create Your Healthy-Eating Plan.* Mayo Clinic. https://www.mayoclinic.org/diseases-conditions/diabetes/in-depth/diabetes-diet/art-20044295#:~:text=If%20you%20have%20diabetes%20or,control%20heart%20disease%20risk%20factors.%5C

Diabetes An♦ Healthy Eating. Better Health. https://www.betterhealth.vic.gov.au/health/conditionsandtreatments/diabetes-and-healthy-eating

Made in the USA
Columbia, SC
11 December 2024

48905245R00111